I0094451

THE ULTIMATE GUIDE
TO CANCER SUPPORT
FOR PATIENTS AND CAREGIVERS

Where to find and access support, information
and resources for a better cancer journey

A COMPANION TO
SURVIVE AND THRIVE!
HOW CANCER SAVES LIVES

Australia
Canada
Ireland
New Zealand
UK
USA

Jo Spicer

CROWN KENT

Copyright © 2019 Jo Spicer

Published by Crown Kent
www.crownkent.com

In accordance with the U.S. Copyright Act of 1976, and the Australian
Copyright Act of 1968, the scanning, uploading, and electronic sharing of any
part of this book without the permission of the publisher constitutes unlawful
piracy and theft of the author's intellectual property. If you would like to
use material from the book (other than for review purposes), prior written
permission must be obtained from the publisher at crownkent.com. Thank you
for your support of the author's rights.

ISBN: 978-0-6484361-1-9

Disclaimer:
The information and opinions expressed in this book are based only on the
personal experience of the author. The author is not a medical practitioner of
any kind and the book is not intended as a medical guide or manual. It is not
designed to provide diagnosis or treatment or any type of professional medical
advice. If you or any other individual chooses to take any recommendations
from this book, please do not do so before consulting your health care
professionals. The list is current at the time of publishing and includes as many
groups and organisations as could be identified. To provide updates or new
inclusions, please email the author: info@jospicer.com

Dedicated to patients and caregivers,
family and friends, affected by cancer.
May this resource and workbook empower
you to create a better cancer journey.

The Survive and Thrive!
SERIES

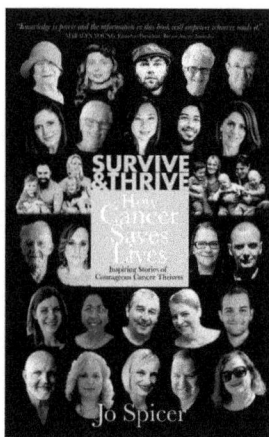

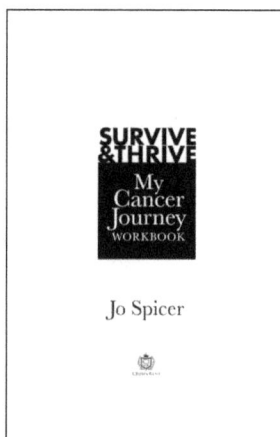

For your FREE download of

Survive and Thrive! My Cancer Journey Workbook

and Jo's other books, go to:

www.jospicer.com

Contents

Introduction

While writing Survive and Thrive! How Cancer Saves Lives, many of the people I interviewed discussed the role of support organisations in their recovery of both body and mind.

It was not only the services and resources that these groups provided, but also the kindness and care of the people they met through these organisations. Many of these people are volunteers, dedicating their time and energy to assist patients. Some of these new connections resulted in lasting friendships. In other cases, mentorship and association with others who had similar diagnoses also proved to be beneficial.

With this in mind, I created this resource to enable all cancer patients and caregivers to find and access the services and support they need during diagnosis, treatment, recovery and beyond.

This book is divided into three parts. Part One briefly summarises the chapters for patients and caregivers in Survive and Thrive! How Cancer Saves Lives.

Part Two is a directory of cancer support organisations and groups in Australia, New Zealand, USA, Canada, the UK and Ireland. The list is current at the time of publishing and includes as many as could be located.

Part Three is my gift to help patients and primary caregivers to stay on track, especially when life is in turmoil and important details and information can get lost. My Cancer Journey Workbook is the place to record doctors' visits, medication, treatment protocols and more. Use it to ensure that these vital notes are all stored in one place for easy reference.

For every person who offers their assistance and time through support organisations and groups, we thank you. For anyone who needs help on their own cancer journey or with caring for a loved one, I hope this book assists you in accessing exactly what you need to survive and thrive.

Jo Spicer

For the Patient

How to cope with your Cancer Diagnosis

Being diagnosed with cancer is possibly one of the scariest things that can ever happen to a person. It is the unknown that makes us fearful, so here are some tips to help you find your way.

1. **Ask questions**

   There is no limit to the number of questions you can ask. Research what you have been told and ask your medical team specific questions to help you understand what treatment they are proposing.

2. **Find the right medical fit**

   Doctors are highly trained humans. Not everyone connects well with each other, and doctors with the same title may have differing opinions. There is nothing wrong with getting a second opinion. Work with a medical team with whom you are happy and confident.

3. **Emotional trauma**

   There is no right or wrong way to react to a cancer diagnosis. Whatever you feel, your emotions are valid.

4. **Find a guide/mentor/counsellor**

   Reach out to a friend, support group or organisation to connect with someone who has overcome a similar diagnosis, or someone with whom you can talk freely. This will help you to mentally and emotional process your situation.

5. **Choose a support person**

   This person will be your primary caregiver. It may be your partner, parent, sibling or good friend. This person will be someone who is happy to walk through your entire journey with you.

6. Gather your tribe

Identify the people you will bring close during your journey, the ones who will uplift you and support you no matter what.

7. Deal with practicalities

Once you have the information about your treatment, attend to the planning and practicalities by making arrangements for the time you will be out of action. Speak to your employer or business partners and arrange time off. Ensure you have your will, power of attorney, enduring guardianship and advanced care directive in place.

8. Take care of your mind

Taking care of your emotional and mental state throughout your journey is a key part of your positive prognosis. Consider meditation, journaling, writing a blog, enjoying plenty of laughter and positivity.

For the Primary Support Person

How to Be a Great Caregiver

As the primary caregiver, there are things that you can do to make the patient's journey easier.

Be there

Just being available to your loved one and providing a safe place for them to be honest about how they feel and what they need, is priceless.

Be positive

The person diagnosed with cancer is often more worried about their caregiver than they are about themselves. If you can be positive and they can see that you are coping, then that will allow them to transfer their mental energy from worrying about you to the important task of healing.

Be the gatekeeper

Help the patient focus on their recovery by handling things like bills and errands so that they can focus on recovery. Only let through things that will assist your loved one to heal.

Be a researcher

Help your loved one by researching and finding anything you can to help with treatment and support.

How to Cope as a Caregiver

It is totally normal to feel helpless, worried, anxious and overwhelmed by the extra load of caring for a loved one. As a caregiver, you need to look after yourself to ensure that you are able to handle the situation. Here are some tips to help you to "put on your oxygen mask first" so that you can provide the support that your loved one needs.

Mentor/Counsellor

Find someone, a professional or friend who you can talk to about what you are experiencing and to keep you mentally and emotionally well.

Journal/Blog

Write a journal of your thoughts to help you process the situation.

Wellbeing

Keep yourself healthy by making good eating choices, getting enough sleep, exercising and staying grounded.

Accept Help

If friends and family are offering help, accept it in whatever form it comes.

Seek Help

If you do not have a network of friends and family, reach out to the many support organisations and groups in this book. You will discover a world of caring people who can provide what you need.

For Friends and Family

How to Provide Meaningful Support

What can you do to provide meaningful support to someone facing cancer?

Treat them the same

They are a person who has cancer, cancer has not transformed them into a "cancer being". Even though they may not feel well or be able to do things as they used to, they are still the same person so don't be awkward.

Be real

There is no need to say, "You'll be fine," or "You look great!" Just be genuine and willing to listen without judgement.

Offer assistance

One of the best ways you can help is to provide assistance with the daily tasks that are now difficult. Things like childcare, home-cooked meals, transport to appointments and household chores are much appreciated.

Australia

A

AUSTRALIA

Advanced Breast Cancer Group

A unique service that offers women all over Queensland an opportunity to meet and talk with other women on how to manage their illness and treatment, and to answer questions on how to live with the disease.
Web: http://www.advancedbreastcancergroup.org.au
Ph: (07) 3217 2998

Amazon Heart

Meeting the needs of women living with breast cancer through a unique approach to peer support by organising life changing adventures that help women come to terms with their breast cancer experiences and move on to live life fully.
Web: www.amazonheart.org

Andrology Australia

Information and resources for men's health including prostate and testicular cancer.
Web: www.andrologyaustralia.org
Ph: 1300 303 878

ANZUP

An Australian and New Zealand cancer-cooperative clinical trials group that brings together all of the professional disciplines and groups involved in researching and treating urogenital and prostate cancers.
Web: www.anzup.org.au
Ph: (02) 9562 5042

Aussie Breast Cancer Forum

For those affected by breast cancer and their families, friends, carers and loved ones.
Web: www.bcaus.org.au

Australia New Zealand Gynaecological Oncology Group

Improving life for women in Australia and New Zealand through cancer research. Access to clinical trials, support and information.
Web: www.anzgog.org.au
Ph: (02) 8071 4880

Australian Breast Cancer Research

Focused on the prevention, detection, management and treatment of breast cancer to reduce the impact that breast cancer has on Australian families.
Web: www.abcr.com.au
Ph: (08) 8445 2453

Australian Cancer Research Foundation

A foundation with a mission to outsmart cancer by providing world-class scientists with the equipment they need to improve prevention, diagnosis and treatment of all types of cancer.
Web: www.acrf.com.au
Ph: (02) 9223 7833

Australian Cervical Cancer Foundation

Dedicated to creating awareness of cervical cancer and its prevention in Australia through community awareness and school awareness programs. Supports women and their families who are affected by cervical cancer.
Web: www.accf.org.au
Ph: 1300 727 630

Australian Lions Childhood Cancer Research Foundation

A prime focus of increasing survival rates of childhood cancer by supporting cancer research efforts in Australia and around the world.
Web: www.alccrf.lions.org.au

Australian Melanoma Research Foundation

A foundation founded for the purpose of funding research into a cure for melanoma and providing education and awareness of its risks.
Web: www.melanomaresearch.com.au
Ph: 0419 822 969

Australian Prostate Cancer

Established to assist with funding of vital medical research into the detection and treatment of prostate cancer, as well as preventing the metastatic spread of the disease.
Web: www.ausprostatecancer.com.au
Ph: (08) 8243 1101

Australasian Lymphology Association

Aims to provide education and support in the prevention, detection, diagnosis and management of lymphoedema.
Web: www.lymphoedema.org.au
Ph: 1300 935 33

Beyond Five

Committed to improving the quality of life of everyone affected by head and neck cancer through education and access to support. Has a mission to raise awareness of head and neck cancer nationally.
Web: www.beyondfive.org.au
Ph: (02) 8598 8514

Bladder Cancer Australia Charity Foundation

Established to increase public awareness of bladder cancer and to gain support from government. Aims to save lives and reduce costs through campaigning for early detection.
Web: www.bladdercancer.org.au

Bowel Cancer Australia

The leading community-funded charity dedicated to prevention, early diagnosis, research, quality treatment and the best care for everyone affected by bowel cancer.
Web: www.bowelcanceraustralia.org
Ph: 1800 555 494

Brainchild Foundation

Established by medical professionals and dedicated parents and friends to heighten awareness surrounding the huge burden that brain and spinal cord tumours cause to children and their families.
Web: www.brainchild.org.au

Brain Tumour Ahoy

Provides support and information for those living with brain tumours. Raising awareness through merchandise and talking to communities.
Web: www.braintumourahoy.org

Brain Tumour Alliance Australia

The only national brain tumour patient and caregiver organisation in Australia.
Web: www.btaa.org.au
Ph: 1800 857 221

Braver Stronger Smarter

Fighting childhood cancer by raising community and government awareness of the need for better treatments for childhood cancer. Empowering others to become involved and make a difference to children fighting cancer.
Web: www.braverstrongersmarter.org.au
Ph: 0428 252 113

BCI Westmead Breast Cancer Institute

A leading and dynamic organisation in the diagnosis and treatment of breast cancer. Their vision of supporting women with breast cancer today and every day is realised through a multidisciplinary approach linking screening, treatment and clinical care.
Web: www.bci.org.au
Ph: (02) 8890 6728

Breast Aware Australia

With a focus on prevention, this organisation provides education relating to lifestyle, diet, exercise and regular breast checks to minimise the risks of women developing breast cancer through early detection.
Web: www.breastawareaustralia.com.au

Breast Cancer Care WA

Personalised emotional, practical and financial support for people affected by breast cancer.
Web: www.breastcancer.org.au
Ph: (08) 9324 3703

Breast Cancer Network Australia

A network of more than 120,000 members who work tirelessly to ensure that every Australian diagnosed with breast cancer receives the very best support, information, treatment and care.
Web: www.bcna.org.au
Ph: 1800 500 258

Breast Cancer Trials

A group of world-leading breast cancer doctors and researchers based in Australia and New Zealand committed to exploring and finding better treatments for people affected by breast cancer through clinical trials research.
Web: www.breastcancertrials.org.au
Ph: 1800 423 444
Ph: (02) 4925 3022

Camp Quality

A children's cancer charity that provides innovative programs to develop life skills and strengthen the well-being of children aged 0 – 13 growing up with cancer, and their families.
Web: www.campquality.org.au
Ph: (02) 9876 0500

Can Assist: Cancer Assistance Network

Can Assist is committed to ensuring that all people, regardless of where they live, have access to cancer treatment and care by providing accommodation, financial assistance and practical support to people from rural and regional areas.
Web: www.canassist.com.au
Ph: 1300 226 277
Ph: (02) 9223 9528

CancerAid

A cancer management and support app. Helps cancer patients to personalise their cancer treatment information and also includes a journey organiser.
Web: www.canceraid.com
Ph: 0429 724 428

Cancer Australia

Established by the Australian Government to benefit all Australians affected by cancer, and their families and caregivers. Aims to reduce the impact of cancer and improve the wellbeing of people affected by cancer.
Web: www.canceraustralia.gov.au
Ph: 1800 624 973

Cancer Care Centre

A community-based organisation providing complementary care services in the support of people affected by cancer.
Web: www.cancercareaustralia.org.au
Ph: (08 8272 2411

Cancer Council Australia

An Australian charity that works across every area of every cancer, from research to prevention and support. They help people from the point of diagnosis through to treatment and survivorship.
Phone Support 13 11 20

Australian Capital Territory
Web: www.actcancer.org   Ph: (02) 6257 9999
New South Wales
Web: www.cancercouncil.com.au   Ph: (02) 9334 1900
Northern Territory
Web: www.cancercouncilnt.com.au   Ph: (08) 8927 4888
Queensland
Web: www.cancerqld.org.au   Ph: (07) 3634 5100
South Australia
Web: www.cancersa.org.au   Ph: (08) 8291 4111
Tasmania
Web: www.cancertas.org.au   Ph: (03) 6169 1900
Victoria
Web: www.cancervic.org.au   Ph: (03) 9514 6100
Western Australia
Web: www.cancerwa.asn.au   Ph: (08) 9212 4333

The Cancer Information & Support Society

An open and unbiased source of information and support for people with cancer in Australia. Provides information, support and counselling, promotes freedom of choice in therapies.
Web: www.ciss.org.au
Ph: (02) 9906 2189

Cancer Institute NSW

Working across the health care system to lessen the impact of cancer by promoting better cancer prevention, early detection, diagnosis, treatment and care.

Web: www.cancer.nsw.gov.au
Ph: (02) 8374 5600

Cancer Voices Australia

An independent, 100% volunteer voice of the people affected by cancer. Working to improve the cancer experience for Australians, their families and friends. Active in the areas of diagnosis, information, treatment, research, support, care, survivorship and policy. Working with decision-makers to ensure the patient perspective is heard.

Web: www.cancervoicesaustralia.org

CanTeen

An organisation set up by a group of young cancer patients to help young people cope with cancer in their family. Focuses on helping young cancer patients to deal with their feelings about cancer, connect with other young people and to provide specialist, youth-specific treatment teams.

Web: www.canteen.org.au
Ph: 1800 835 932

Carer Gateway

Information on how to care for someone with cancer.

Web: www.carergateway.gov.au

Challenge

Supporting children diagnosed with cancer and their families with a full range of free programs and services both in and out of hospital.

Web: www.challenge.org.au

Childhood Cancer Association

Provide practical, hands-on support to children with cancer and their families.

Web: www.childhoodcancer.asn.au
Ph: (08) 8239 1444

Childhood Cancer Support

Provide ongoing support for children undergoing cancer treatment by providing a place to call home during treatment, emotional and financial support, transport and recreational therapies.
Web: www.ccs.org.au
Ph: (07) 3844 5000

Children's Cancer Foundation

Enables children with cancer to access the world's best treatment and support. Builds awareness of childhood cancer in the community and within governments. Supports families through treatment. Partners with hospitals to deliver clinical excellence.
Web: www.childrenscancerfoundation.com.au
Ph: (03) 7001 1450

Children's Cancer Institute

Operate with a vision to save the lives of all children with cancer and improve their long-term health, through research.
Web: www.ccia.org.au
Ph: 1800 685 686

Children's Leukaemia & Cancer Research Foundation

Raising funds to ensure that research continues to find cures so that future generations will live cancer free.
Web: www.childcancerresearch.com.au
Ph: (08) 9363 7400

Children's Medical Research Institute

A mission to find cures for children's genetic diseases.
Web: www.cmri.org.au
Ph: 1800 436 437
Ph: (02) 8865 2800

Chris O'Brien Lifehouse

Lifehouse is an integrated and focused centre of excellence, offering everything a cancer patient needs in one place, including advanced onco-surgery, chemotherapy, radiation therapy, clinical trials, research, education, complementary therapies and psychosocial support.
Web: www.mylifehouse.org.au
Ph: 1300 852 500

Counterpoint
Connects, supports and informs women living with breast or a gynaecological cancer to live well. Access to trained peer support volunteers with lived experience of cancer.
Web: www.counterpart.org.au
Ph: 1300 781 500

Country Hope Trust
Provides family centred support services to country children diagnosed with cancer and other life-threatening illnesses.
Web: www.countryhope.com.au
Ph: 1800 007 880
Ph: (02) 6971 8955

Cure Brain Cancer Foundation
Australia's leading organisation for brain cancer research, advocacy and awareness. A strong patient focus bringing world-class clinical trials to Australia to give children and adults with brain cancer access to new treatments faster.
Web: www.curebraincancer.org.au
Ph: (02) 8973 1400

Cure Cancer Australia
Funding crucial cancer research from Australia's brightest emerging minds. Investing in innovators in cancer research who offer new ideas and challenging perspectives to advance the fight against all types of cancer.
Web: www.curecancer.com.au
Ph: (02) 8072 6188

Dragons Abreast
Encourages wellness, fitness, fun and camaraderie for breast cancer survivors through the sport of dragon boating. Promotes breast cancer awareness throughout the community.
Web: www.dragonsabreast.com.au
Ph: 1300 889 566

Dreams 2 Live 4

Making dreams come true for patients who are living with metastatic cancer.

Web: www.dreams2live4.com.au

Ph: 0400 914 375

F

Fight Cancer Foundation

A national charity providing care, treatment and support for cancer patients and their families and funding vital research into cancer treatment and cures. Established Australia's first bone marrow donor registry and has now broadened its scope to providing support services for patients with blood and other cancers.

Web: www.fightcancer.org.au

Ph: (03) 93427888

G

The Gawler Cancer Foundation

An active cancer support group created by cancer survivor, Ian Gawler. Teaches people how to increase their chances of survival and improve quality of life.

Web: www.gawler.org

Ph: (03) 5967 1730

GI Cancer

Conducting research and clinical trials to save and improve the lives of patients with gastro-intestinal (GI) cancer.

Web: www.gicancer.org.au

Ph: 1300 666 769

I

Inspire

A support and discussion community for Appendix Cancer – Pseudomyxoma Peritonei Cancer.

Web: www.inspire.com

AUSTRALIA

K

AUSTRALIA

Kidney Cancer On-Line Support

A cooperative site intended for support and sharing of information between kidney cancer sufferers.
Web: www.akcos.org

Kidney Health Australia

Dedicated to helping people with kidney disease, with a view to improving their health outcomes and quality of life, and that of their families and carers.
Web: www.kidney.org.au
Ph: 1800 454 363

The Kids' Cancer Project

This organisation stands for science, solutions and survival.
Web: www.thekidscancerproject.org.au
Ph: 1800 651 158

Kids Cancer Support Group

Connecting, supporting and enriching the lives of kids diagnosed with cancer and other blood disorders.
Web: www.kcsg.org.au
Ph: 0438 878 622

Kids with Cancer Foundation Australia

Helping struggling families of kids with cancer and the children's hospitals where they are treated.
Web: www.kidswithcancer.org.au
Ph: 1800 255 522

Koala Kids

A volunteer-driven organisation that provides therapeutic resources, family support and entertaining activities in Children's Cancer Centres.
Web: www.koalakids.org.au
Ph: (03) 8589 4812

AUSTRALIA

Leila Rose Foundation
Offers support and guidance to families when faced with childhood cancer. Assistance from diagnosis and throughout treatment to help them feel empowered to make informed decisions about their child's health.
Web: www.leilarosefoundation.org

Leukaemia Foundation
A national charity dedicated to helping those with leukaemia, lymphoma, myeloma and related blood disorders to survive and then live a better quality of life.
Web: www.leukaemia.org.au
Ph: 1800 620 420

Little Heroes
Supports seriously ill children and their families with essential equipment and services.
Web: www.littleheroesfoundation.com.au
Ph: (08) 7099 3628

Look Good Feel Better
Teaching cancer patients how to manage the appearance-related side-effects caused by cancer treatment. Women, men and teens participate in a practical workshop which covers skincare, make-up and headwear demonstrations leaving them empowered and ready to face their cancer diagnosis with confidence.
Web: www.lgfb.org.au
Ph: 1800 650 960

Lung Foundation Australia
Working to improve lung health and reduce the impact of lung disease for all Australians. Supporting people of all ages with lung disease at every stage of their journey.
Web: www.lungfoundation.com.au
Ph: 1800 654 301

Lymphoma Australia
Supports lymphoma research, patients and families. Funds lymphoma care nurses and raises awareness of the signs and symptoms for earlier diagnosis.
Web: www.lymphoma.org.au
Ph: 1800 359 081

Make-A-Wish Foundation

The power of a single wish can change lives. By giving seriously ill children a chance to escape their reality and just focus on being a kid, this foundation helps them to regain hope.
Web: www.makeawish.org.au
Ph: 1800 032 260

McGrath Foundation

A foundation raising money to fund McGrath Breast Care Nurses in communities across Australia who help individuals and families experiencing breast cancer by providing physical, psychological and emotional support for free.
Web: www.mcgrathfoundation.com.au
Ph: (02) 8962 6100

Melanoma Institute Australia

Pioneers advances in melanoma research and treatment. A national affiliated network of melanoma researchers and clinicians based at the Poche Centre Sydney, the world's largest melanoma research and treatment facility where they run clinical trials and treat 1,500 melanoma patients each year.
Web: www.melanoma.org.au
Ph: (02) 9911 7200

Melanoma Patients Australia

An independent organisation supporting those affected by melanoma. Services include counselling, education, peer-to-peer connections and support groups delivered face-to-face, by phone and online.
Web: www.melanomapatients.org.au
Ph: 1300 884 450

The Movember Foundation

Focussed on changing the face of men's health addressing prostate cancer, testicular cancer, mental health and suicide prevention.
Web: www.movember.com.au
Ph: 1300 4769 66

AUSTRALIA

Myeloma Foundation

Facilitates myeloma research in Australia. Supports and informs those living with the disease and educate those involved in its care and treatment.
Web: www.myeloma.org.au
Ph: (03) 9428 7444

My Room

A volunteer organisation dedicated to raising funds to achieve a 100% cure rate for childhood cancers. Supports research, clinical care and families to improve the quality of life for children with cancer.
Web: www.myroom.com.au

N

National Breast Cancer Foundation

Australia's leading national body funding world, game-changing breast cancer research.
Web: www.nbcf.org.au

Neuroblastoma Australia

Raising funds so that children with all types of neuroblastoma survive and lead long, healthy lives, free from the side-effects of their treatment.
Web: www.neuroblastoa.org.au
Ph: 0406 991 606

O

Olivia Newton-John Cancer Wellness and Research Centre

A multidisciplinary approach to ensure that cancer patients are cared for physically, psychologically, emotionally and spiritually. Committed to providing support through every step of treatment and beyond.
Web: www.onjcancercentre.org
Ph: (03) 9496 5000

Otis Foundation

A charity that provides a national network of retreat accommodation properties at no cost to anyone who has faced the challenge of breast cancer.
Web: www.otisfoundation.org.au
Ph: (03) 5444 1185

Ovarian Cancer Australia
Founded with the vision to save lives and ensures that no woman
with ovarian cancer walk alone. Works with the community to raise
awareness. Provides support face-to-face, over the phone or online.
Web: www.ovariancancer.net.au
Ph: 1300 660 334

Pancare Foundation
Support services for pancreatic and other upper gastrointestinal cancers.
Providers of financial aid and emotional support with a dedicated
community care program.
Web: www.pancare.org.au
Ph: 1300 881 698

Peter MacCallum Cancer Centre
Assist patients and their families and carers with the physical, emotional
and financial impacts of a cancer diagnosis. Incorporates the Australian
Cancer Survivorship Centre.
Web: www.petermac.org
Ph: (03) 8559 5000

Prostate Cancer Foundation of Australia
A broad-based community organisation dedicated to reducing the
impact of prostate cancer on Australian men, their partners and
families.
Web: www.prostate.org.au
Ph: 1800 22 00 99

Pink Hope
Provides the community with personalised support, information and
resources including a genetic counsellor, online support group and
health and education days.
Web: www.pinkhope.org.au
Ph: (02) 8084 2288

Q

Quest for Life Foundation
Established by Petrea King, the foundation provides practical skills and strategies for people to create peace and resilience for their lives.
Web: www.questforlife.com.au
Ph: 1300 941 488

R

Redkite
Providers of essential support to children and young people (aged up to 24) with cancer, and their families. Support services from diagnosis, throughout and after treatment.
Web: www.redkite.org.au
Ph: 1800 733 548

S

AUSTRALIA

Sisters' Cancer Support Group
The first multicultural specific cancer support group registered with Cancer Council NSW and Breast Cancer Network Australia. Working to support women from multicultural communities affected by cancer.
Web: www.scsg.or.au
Ph: 0415 238 990

South Australian Prostate Cancer Clinical Outcome Collaboration
A multi-centre, multidisciplinary collaboration between men diagnosed with prostate cancer to create a comprehensive collection of data to better understand the disease. Has helpful information to assist in dealing with the disease and life after treatment.
Web: www.prostatehealth.org.au
Ph: (08) 8204 7672

Starlight Children's Foundation
Replaces pain, fear and stress with fun joy and laughter for sick children and their families. Providing programs that are impactful and of real value to the lives of sick kids, their families and health professionals.
Web: www.starlight.org.au
Ph: 1300 727 827

Telethon Kids Institute

Intent on building a research institute that makes a real difference in the community, benefiting children and families everywhere.

Web: www.telethonkids.org.au

Ph: (08) 6319 1000

Tour de Cure

Riding to Cure Cancer. Raising funds to support doctors and scientists who have dedicated their lives to uncovering a cure.

Web: www.tourdecure.com.au

Ph: (02) 8073 4000

Unicorn Foundation

Seeking the cure for neuroendocrine cancers (NETS). They assist and support patients and carers; lobby for new, appropriate treatments and investigations; raise awareness and knowledge of NETS.

Web: www.unicornfoundation.org.au

Ph: 1300 287 363

YWCA Encore

Helping women with the after-effects of breast cancer surgery and treatment. Helping to restore strength, mobility and flexibility, confidence and general wellbeing through a free eight-week program of specially designed exercise, support and information.

Web: www.ywcaencore.org.au

Ph: 1800 305 150

Ph: (02) 9285 6264

Canada

B

C
A
N
A
D
A

Bladder Cancer Canada

Devoted to awareness, support and research to create a world where bladder cancer is just a memory.
Web: www.bladdercancercanada.org
Ph: 866 674 8889

Brain Tumour Foundation of Canada

A dedicated team of volunteers, patients, survivors, family members, health care professionals and staff, determined to make the journey with a brain tumour one full of hope and support.
Web: www.braintumour.ca
Ph: 1800 265 5106

C

Canadian Breast Cancer Network

Canada's leading patient-directed organisation of individuals striving to voice the views and concerns of breast cancer patients through education, advocacy activities and the promotion of information sharing.
Web: www.cbcn.ca
Ph: 1 800 685 8820
Ph: 613 230 3044

Canadian Cancer Society

A national, community-based organisation of volunteers whose mission is the eradication of cancer and the enhancement of the quality of life of people living with cancer.
Web: www.cancer.ca
Ph: 888 939 3333
Ph: 519 642 7755

Canadian Cancer Survivor Network

Promoting health by conducting educational activities for cancer patients, caregivers and survivors.
Web: www.survivornet.ca
Ph: 613 898 1871v

Cancer Advocacy Coalition Canada

An effective, comprehensive, evidence-based cancer system that offers Canadians the best chance for preventing and treating cancer. Addresses the emotional, physical and financial needs of patients and survivors.
Web: www.anceradvocacy.ca
Ph: 1 855 572 3436
Ph: 416 642 6472

Cancer Chat Canada

Professionally-led online support groups for Canadians affected by cancer, including patients, survivors and family members.
Web: www.cancerchat.desouzainstitute.com

Cancertainty

A united voice for high-quality cancer treatment for all patients regardless of age, income or postal code.
Web: wwwlcancertaintyforall.ca
Ph: 647 290 7573

Carcinoid-Neuroendocrine Tumour Society Canada

Patient education, webinars, conferences, resources and support for patients with neuroendocrine tumours.
Web: www.cnetscanada.org
Ph: 1844 628 6788

Childhood Cancer Canada

Offers vital programs to help and educate families such as emPower Pack, Amazing Adventures, Survivor Scholarships and Benevolent Fund. A strong focus on saving, enhancing and extending the lives of kids with cancer.
Web: www.childhoodcancer.ca
Ph: 1800 363 1062

Colorectal Cancer Canada

Dedicated to increasing awareness of colorectal cancer, supporting patients, and advocating on their behalf.
Web: www.coloretalcancercanada.com
Ph: 887 502 6566
Ph: 613 730 4192

Coping With Cancer

Created to support patients, families and caregivers to find clarity and to start down the path of coping with cancer.
Web: www.copingwithcancer.ca
Ph: 416 968 0207

Hereditary Breast and Ovarian Cancer Society

Representing, educating and supporting individuals, families and communities affected by HBOC syndrome.
Web: www.hbocsociety.org
Ph: 780 488 4262
Ph: 866 786 4262

HopeSprings

An independent community organisation committed to empowering those whose lives are impacted by cancer. Aims to improve their emotional, physical and spiritual wellbeing.
Web: www.hopesprings.ca
Ph: 519 742 4673

I Had Cancer

A cancer support community that empowers people to take control of life before, during and after cancer. This peer-to-peer support is crucial in allowing survivors, fighters and supporters/caregivers to share first hand experiences about treatment, side-effects, long-term effects and more.
Web: www.ihadcancer.com

Island Prostate Centre

Supporting Vancouver Island men and their families at every step of their journey through diagnosis, decision, treatment and recovery from prostate cancer.
Web: www.islandprostatecentre.com
Ph: 1 866 388 0214
Ph: 250 388 0214

K

C
A
N
A
D
A

Kidney Cancer Association Canada

A charitable organisation comprising patients, family members, physicians, researchers and other health professionals globally. It is the world's first international charity dedicated specifically to the eradication of death and suffering from renal cancers.
Web: www.kidneycancer.org
Ph: 403 800 3112

Kidney Cancer Canada

A national community of patients, caregivers and health professionals who work to provide support, education and advocacy for the care pathways and treatment options of any Canadian touched by kidney cancer.
Web: www.kidneycancercanada.ca
Ph: 1 866 598 7166

L

The Leukaemia/Bone Marrow Transplant Program of BC

Providing patients, families, physicians and health care workers with extensive information about the Leukaemia/Bone Marrow Transplant Program of British Columbia.
Web: www.leukemiabmtprogram.org
Ph: 604 875 4343

Leukaemia & Lymphoma Society of Canada

A mission to cure leukaemia, lymphoma, Hodgkin's disease and myeloma and to improve the quality of life for patients and their families through research, patient support and advocacy.
Web: www.llscanada.org
Ph: 877 668 8326

Look Good, Feel Better

A site for teens with cancer. Look good, feel better website for teenager, answering questions that teens with cancer ask.
Web: www.lgfb.ca

Lung Cancer Canada

Canada's leading resource for lung cancer education and support.
Web: www.lungcancercanada.ca
Ph: 416 785 3439

Lymphoma Canada

Supports and promotes support groups across the country. Empowering lymphoma patients and the lymphoma community through support, education and research.
Web: www.lymphoma.ca
Ph: 905 858 5967

Melanoma Network of Canada

Founded to respond to the need for Canada to have a nationally-based organisation to coordinate education and prevention efforts, provide a strong voice for advocacy and assist in efforts to target funding for melanoma research.
Web: www.melanomanetwork.ca
Ph: 1 877 560 8035

Multiple Myeloma Vancouver Island Support Group

Offering education and assistance to all those touched by myeloma by sharing information, concerns and successes.
Web: www.myelomavancouverisland.ca

My Gut Feeling

Peer support, awareness and education for patients, survivors and caregivers affected by stomach cancer.
Web: www.mygutfeeling.ca
Ph: 647 478 5414

Ovarian Cancer Canada

Supporting women living with ovarian cancer, raising awareness and funding research.
Web: www.ovariancanada.org
Ph: 1 877 413 7970

Pancreatic Cancer Canada

Fighting cancer on all fronts: research, awareness, community activation and advocacy.
Web: www.pancreaticcancercanada.ca
Ph: 1 888 726 2269
Ph: 416 548 8077

Prostate Cancer Foundation
Volunteers working tirelessly to support men and their families in BC.
Providing events programs and services to support and educate.
Web: www.prostatecancerbc.ca
Ph: 604 574 4012
Ph: 1 877 840 9173

Saskatchewan Cancer Agency
Operates prevention and early detection programs, conducts innovative
research and provides safe, patient and family-centred care.
Web: www.saskcancer.ca
Ph: 639 625 2010

The Society of Obstetricians and Gynaecologists of Canada
Evidence-based information about HPV. Resources and educational
information to answer your questions about this disease.
Web: www.hpvinfo.ca
Ph: 800 561 2416

Starlight Children's Foundation Canada
Creating moments of joy and comfort to hospitalised children and their
families. For 35 years, Starlight has brought smiles to more than 60
million critically, chronically and terminally ill children in the United
States, Canada, Australia and the United Kingdom.
Web: www.starlightcanada.org

Testicular Cancer Canada
Increasing awareness, providing information and support for men who
have testicular cancer.
Web: www.testicularcancer.ngo
Ph: 416 628 3189

Thyroid Cancer Canada
A national organisation of thyroid cancer survivors dedicated to
providing emotional support and information to those affected by the
disease.
Web: www.thyroidcancercanada.org
Ph: 416 487 8267

Wellspring

Improves the quality of life for people living with cancer from diagnosis, through treatment and into survivorship, helping them overcome emotional, social and practical challenges.
Web: www.wellspring.ca

Calgary Ph: 403 521 5292

Edmonton Ph: 780 758 4433

Toronto Ph: 416 961 1928

Sunnybrook Ph: 416 480 4440

London Ph: 519 438 7379

Niagara Ph: 905 684 7619

Stratford Ph: 519 271 2232

Brampton Ph: 905 792 6480

Oakville Ph: 905 257 1988

Young Adult Cancer Canada

A network of hundreds of young adults affected by cancer. Supports young adults as they live with, through and beyond cancer. Facilitates connection to peers, builds bridges out of isolation and inspiration.
Web: www.youngadultcancer.ca

Ireland

ARC Cancer Support

Support, complementary therapies and counselling services in a warm and welcoming environment to people with cancer and those who care for them.
Web: www.arccancersupport.ie
Eccles St Ph: 01 830 7333
South Circular Rd Ph: 01 707 8880

Brain Tumour Ireland

Supports brain tumour patients with meetings in Dublin, Cork and Galway.
Web: www.braintumourireland.com
Ph: 074 96 01901

Cancer Care West

Professional community-based practical and emotional support services to anyone affected by cancer.
Web: www.cancercarewest.ie
Galway Ph: 091 540 040
Donegal Ph: 074 960 1901
University Hospital Ph: 091 545 000

Cancer Support Sanctuary

Offers psychological and emotional support to people living with cancer, providing a homely environment where patients and family members can engage in services including one-on-one counselling, complementary therapies, nurse support and classes.
Web: www.cancersupport.ie
Ph: 1 850 719 719

CanTeen Ireland

A nationwide support group for young people between the ages of 12 and 25 years old who have had cancer.
Web: www.canteen.ie
Ph: 01 872 2012

IRELAND

Childhood Cancer Foundation

Supporting Irelands fight against cancer. A resource to connect families to support groups.
Web: www.childhoodcancer.ie
Ph: 1 554 5655

Cork ARC Cancer Support House

A safe haven for people with cancer and their families. Information, practical help and emotional support.
Web: www.corkcancersupport.ie
Ph: 021 427 6688

E

EIST Cancer Support Centre Carlow

Therapies, counselling, support, classes and workshops for people affected by cancer.
Web: www.eistcarlcancersupport.ie
Ph: 059 913 9684

G

Greystones Cancer Support

Counselling, support, therapies and information for people affected by cancer.
Web: www.greystonescancersupport.com
Ph: 01 287 1601

H

Hope Cancer Support Centre

Emotional support and practical information for people whose lives are changed by cancer.
Web: www.hopesupportcentre.ie
Ph: 053 923 8555

I

Irish Cancer Society

Offers on-on-one support. Information and an online community to help anyone affected by cancer.
Web: www.cancer.ie
Ph: 1800 200 700

K

Kerry Cancer Support Group

Devoted to maintaining a warm, welcoming environment to provide cancer patients with immediate access to their programmes and resources.
Web: www.kerrycancersupport.com
Ph: 066 7195560

M

MAC

Men Against Cancer provides non-medical support, counselling and information for men diagnosed with prostate cancer and their families.
Web: www.macprostatecancersupport.ie
Ph: 01 254 2887

Marie Keating Foundation

Free cancer services and support for cancer patients and their families. Support centres located throughout Ireland.
Web: www.mariekeating.ie
Ph: 01 628 3726

Multiple Myeloma Ireland

Solely focused on providing information and support for multiple myeloma patients, families and carers.
Web: www.multiplemyelomaireland.org
Ph: 867 804 007

P

Purple House Cancer Support

Provides cancer support groups, helpline, and survivorship programmes.
Web: www.purplehouse.ie
Ph: 1 286 6966

S

Solas Cancer Support Centre

Offering free cancer support services to the people of Waterford and the South East of Ireland.
Web: www.solascentre.ie
Ph: 51 304 604

IRELAND

T

I
R
E
L
A
N
D

Tallaght Cancer Support Group

Encourages healing of anyone touched by cancer through friendship and support.

Web: www.tallaghtcancersupport.com

Ph: 086 400 2736

New Zealand

ANZUP

An Australian and New Zealand cancer-cooperative clinical trials group that brings together all of the professional disciplines and groups involved in researching and treating urogenital and prostate cancers.
Web: www.anzup.org.au
Ph: +61 2 9562 5042

Aratika Cancer Trust

"Aratika" means "the right path". This trust believes attending to the emotional, mental, spiritual and physical health is essential for wellbeing. They offer workshops and retreats exploring evidence-based integrative medicine practices to educate and empower people with a cancer diagnosis.
Web: www.aratikatrust.co.nz
Ph: 022 429 5063

Aroha Mai Cancer Support Services

A voluntary team extending support services to cancer sufferers and their families through counselling, assistance and education for the Maori and wider community.
Web: www.arohamai.maori.nz
Ph: 07 349 3118

Australia New Zealand Gynaecological Oncology Group

Improving life for women in Australia and New Zealand through cancer research. Access to clinical trials, support and information.
Web: www.anzgog.org.au
Ph: +61 2 8071 4880

Australasian Lymphology Association

Aims to provide education and support in the prevention, detection, diagnosis and management of lymphoedema.
Web: www.lymphoedema.org.au
Ph: 0800 866 030

AYA Cancer Network Aotearoa

Advancing cancer care for those aged 12–24 years. Ensuring all young people diagnosed with cancer in New Zealand have equitable access to high quality medical and supportive care regardless of where they live.
Web: www.ayacancernetwork.org.nz
Ph: 021 337 129

Bowel Cancer New Zealand

A nationwide, patient led organisation committed to reducing the impact of bowel cancer on the community through awareness, education, support and research.
Web: www.beatbowelcancer.org.nz
Ph: 021 027 51924

Bowel & Liver Trust

A charitable trust advancing education and research in gut diseases,
Web: www.bowelandliver.org.nz
Ph: (03) 928 1536

Breast Cancer Aotearoa Coalition

Providing a wide range of support and information to New Zealanders and their families who are experiencing breast cancer.
Web: www.breastcancer.org.nz

Breast Cancer Cure

Established solely to find a cure for breast cancer.
Web: www.breastcancercure.org.nz
Ph: 0800 227 828

Breast Cancer Foundation

Pushing for new frontiers in early detection, treatment and support. Support services for patients, their families and friends.
Web: www.breastcancerfoundation.org.nz
Ph: 0800 902 732

Breast Cancer Northland

Offering practical and emotional support for people diagnosed with breast cancer and living in the Northland region.
Web: www.breastcancernorthland.co.nz
Ph: 0800 227 687

Breast Cancer Support

New Zealand's foremost not-for-profit specialising in peer support services for women experiencing breast cancer.
Web: www.breastcancersupport.co.nz
Ph: 0800 273 222

Breast Cancer Support Service Tauranga

A local independent charitable trust based on the principle of survivors supporting those newly diagnosed. Covering the Western Bay of Plenty.
Web: www.breastcancerbop.org.nz
Ph: (07) 571 3346

Breast Cancer Trials

A group of world-leading breast cancer doctors and researchers based in Australia and New Zealand committed to exploring and finding better treatments for people affected by breast cancer through clinical trials research.
Web: www.breastcancertrials.org.au
Ph: +61 2 4925 3022

Busting With Life

Providing hope and inspiration to those with breast cancer through heightening awareness of breast cancer and by encouraging active living through dragon boat paddling.
Web: www.bustingwithlife.org.nz
Ph: 021 502 351

Cancer Chat

A forum hosted by the Cancer Society for anyone who has been touched by cancer.
Web: www.cancerchatnz.org.nz

NEW ZEALAND

Cancer Society

A comprehensive resource offering emotional support, access to nurses, support groups, home care, complementary and alternative therapies and financial assistance.
Web: www.cancernz.org.nz
Ph: 0800 226 237

Canopy Cancer Care

A private clinic offer world class cancer treatment with chemotherapy, immunotherapy, antibody therapy, hormone therapy and more targeted therapies.
Web: www.canopycancercare.co.nz
Epsom Ph: 09 623 5602
North Shore Ph: 09 623 5602
Tauranga Ph: 07 562 1366

CanTeen

Helping young people touched by cancer to continue living life by providing the support and tools they need.
Web: www.canteen.org.nz
Ph: 09 303 4444

Child Cancer Foundation

Provides strength and comfort to families and children impacted by childhood cancer with personalised emotional, social and practical support.
Web: www.childcancer.org.nz
Ph: (09) 366 1270

Central Cancer Network

Working across organisational boundaries to promote a collaborative approach to reduce the incidence and impact of cancer; to reduce the inequalities with respect to cancer; and to improve the journey of cancer patients and their families.
Web: www.centralcancernetwork.org.nz
Ph: 06 3508918

The Gift of Knowledge
Focused on raising awareness, connecting patients to others, supporting them to make informed decisions, advocating and ultimately contributing to reducing the impact and incidence of hereditary breast and ovarian cancer.
Web: www.giftofknowledge.co.nz
Ph: 021 942 889

Gut Cancer Foundation
Dedicated to improving the outcomes for patients with gastro-intestinal cancer.
Web: www.gutcancer.org.nz
Ph: 0800 112 775

Head and Neck Cancer Survivors Support Network
Created to connect, provide support and advocate for survivors of head and neck cancer.
Web: www.headandneck.org.nz
Ph: 021 213 0178

Kathleen Kilgour Centre
Leaders in Radiation Therapy. Work closely with the Cancer Society to offer complementary services.
Web: www.kathleenkilgourcentre.co.nz
Ph: (07) 929 7995

Kenzie's Gift
Committed to improving the emotional wellbeing and mental health of children, young people and their families through serious illness or bereavement.
Web: www.kenziesgift.com
Ph: 027 345 2514

L

Leukaemia & Blood Cancer New Zealand
A vision to cure and a mission to care. Committed to improving the quality of life for patients and their families living with leukaemia, lymphoma, myeloma and related blood conditions.
Web: www.leukaemia.org.nz
Ph: 0800 15 10 15

Look Good, Feel Better
Teaching cancer patients how to manage the appearance-related side-effects caused by cancer treatment. Women, men and teens participate in a practical workshop which covers skincare, make-up and headwear demonstrations leaving them empowered and ready to face their cancer diagnosis with confidence.
Web: www.lgfb.co.nz
Ph: 0800 865 432

Lymphoedema Support Network
Provides practical information and support to people living with lymphoedema and their families.
Web: www.lyphoedema.org.nz
Ph: 09 625 6463

Lymphoma Network New Zealand
Working to improve patient care lymphoma patients by collaborating and exchanging information in the field of lymphoma.
Web: www.lymphomanetworknz.co.nz

Lung Foundation
Educating and supporting New Zealanders with lung cancer.
Web: www.lungfoundation.org.nz
Ph: 021 959 450

Melanoma NZ
New Zealand's only charity organisation dedicated to preventing avoidable deaths and suffering from melanoma by providing information, regular skin checks for early detection, support and advocacy.
Web: www.melanoma.org.nz
Ph: (09) 449 2342

Melnet
A network of professionals working together to reduce the incidence and impact of melanoma in New Zealand.
Web: www.melnet.org.nz
Ph: 027 492 6650

Mercury Bay Cancer Support Group
Comprised of local volunteers who provide a support network for individuals and families that are affected by cancer in the Whitianga and wider Mercury Bay area.
Web: www.allaboutwhitianga.co.nz/mercury-bay-clubs-organisations/welfare-organisations/mercury-bay-cancer-support-group

Multiple Myeloma
Focused on improving survival, raising awareness and supporting patients with multiple myeloma.
Web: www.multiplemyeloma.org.nz
Ph: 02 744 32624

New Zealand Gynaecological Cancer Foundation
Educating women and the community about the signs and symptoms of gynaecological cancers. A national organisation providing support, advocacy and awareness.
Web: www.nzgcf.org.nz
Ph: 0275 630 147

O

Ovarian Cancer New Zealand
Providing support, awareness and advocacy for those touched by ovarian cancer.
Web: www.ovariancancernz.org.nz

P

N E W   Z E A L A N D

Pinc & Steel
Helping people affected by cancer through physical rehabilitation. Committed to supporting people affected by any type of cancer through all stages of their treatment and recovery. Programs throughout New Zealand including classes, walking, running, biking and more.
Web: www.pinkandsteel.com

Pink Dragons
A group of dynamic breast cancer survivors with a zest for life. Supporting each other through paddling and dragon boat racing regardless of age or athletic ability.
Web: www.pinkdragonsorg.nz

Pink Pilates
Designed to help women diagnosed with cancer to regain their physical strength, improve their body confidence and incorporate exercise into their lives.
Web: www.pinkpilates.co.nz
Ph: 09 304 0969

Prostate Cancer Foundation
A strong focus on promoting public awareness of prostate cancer. Assists with advocacy, research and peer support with 36 support networks across New Zealand.
Web: www.prostate.org.nz
Ph: 0800 477 678

Rotorua Breast Cancer Trust
Supporting and caring for those in their community affected by breast cancer.
Web: www.rotoruabreastcancertrust.co.nz
Ph: 022 424 6616

Shocking Pink
Support groups and services to support young women through breast cancer and beyond.
Web: www.shockingpink.org.nz

Sweet Louise
A single-minded vision of improving the quality of life for New Zealanders living with incurable breast cancer.
Web: www.sweetlouise.co.nz

Taranaki Dragons
A proud, positive and motivated group of women who are committed to leading full and active lives. Aim to promote awareness of breast cancer and survivorship, offer support, make new friendships, increase fitness and have fun along the way.
Web: www.taranakidragons.co.nz
Ph: 027 870 1645

Waikato Breast Cancer Research Trust
Working with international and local research groups to provide New Zealand women with access to improved treatments, reduce side-effects, better communication and quality of life.
Web: www.wbcrt.org.nz
Ph: 07 839 8726

Well Women & Family Trust
Founded to provide clinical services that exceed recommendations and ensure women have access to high quality, free, culturally appropriate, respectful and informed cervical screening. Mandated to promote wellness and reduce the mortality and morbidity of cervical cancers in New Zealand.
Web:www.wons.org.nz
Ph: (09) 846 7886

UK

ACC Support UK

Adrenocortical Cancer Support and information for those diagnosed and affected by ACC.
Web: www.accsupport.org.uk
Ph: 0800 434 6476

Action Bladder Cancer UK

Working to support bladder cancer patients, raise awareness, improve early diagnosis and outcomes and to further research.
Web: www.actionbladdercanceruk.org
Ph: 0300 302 0085

AMMF

Raising awareness throughout the UK and collaborating throughout the world to cure bile duct cancer.
Web: www.ammf.org.uk
Ph: 01279 661 479

Ayrshire Cancer Support

A local charity providing emotional support and practical help to those affected by cancer.
Web: www.ayrshirecs.org
Ayr Ph: 01292 269 888
Kilmarnock Ph: 01563 538 008

Baggy Trousers UK

Aims to raise awareness of testicular cancer in young males as well as providing emotional and financial support, guidance and help for those suffering from testicular cancer.
Web: www.baggytrousersuk.org

Beating Bowel Cancer

Supporting and campaigning for everyone affected by bowel cancer.
Web: www.beatingbowelcancer.org
Ph: 020 8973 0011

Beatson Cancer Charity

Supporting people affected by cancer, every step of the way. Providing services, research and education. Investing in a better future for cancer patients and their families.
Web: www.beatsoncancercharity.org
Ph: 0141 212 0505

Bloodwise

Funding world-class research into all types of blood cancer. Supporting anyone worried about blood cancer with expert information and advice.
Web: www.bloodwise.org.uk
Ph: 0808 2080 888

Bone Cancer Research Trust

Pioneering research into primary bone cancer.
Web: www.bcrt.org.uk
Ph: 0113 258 5934

Bowel Cancer UK

Information, support and resources for everyone affected by bowel cancer.
Web: www.bowelcanceruk.org.uk
Ph: 020 7940 1760

Breast Cancer Care

Provides information, emotional and practical support for those living with breast cancer and beyond.
Web: www.breastcancercare.org.uk
Ph: 0800 800 6000

Breast Cancer Haven

A national organisation offering counselling and therapies to help a woman gain control of her life, treatment and cancer journey.
Web: www.breastcancerhaven.org.uk
London Ph: 020 7384 0099
Hereford Ph: 01432 361 061
Yorkshire Ph: 0113 284 7829
Wessex Ph: 01329 559 290
Worchester Ph: 01905 677 862
West Midlands Ph: 0121 726 9570

U
K

Breast Cancer Now

Organisers of the Wear It Pink awareness campaign. The UK's largest breast cancer research charity.
Web: www.breastcancernow.org
Ph: 0333 20 70 300

The Brain Tumour Charity

A charity providing information and support for anyone affected by brain tumours. Creators of BRIAN (the Brain tumouR Information and Analysis Network). It is an anonymous and secure databank storing the information of people's treatment, tumour types, experiences, side-effects, decision and more to gain insights into all the different types of brain tumour in order to reach a cure quicker.
Web: www.thebraintumourcharity.org
Ph: 0808 800 0004

British Lung Foundation

Connecting lung cancer patients to local support. Information and resources plus access to a helpline to answer questions on symptoms and treatment.
Web: www.blf.org.uk
Ph: 03000 030 555

Butterfly Thyroid Cancer Trust

A national group supporting patients with thyroid cancer. Has a dedicated helpline, connecting group members and a "buddy" to help patients through surgery and treatment.
Web: www.butterfly.org.uk
Ph: 01207 545 467

Cahonas Scotland

Educating men and their partners about testicular, breast and prostate cancers.
Web: www.cahonasscotland.com
Ph: 0141 952 0675

Cancer Care

Helping families affected by cancer in North Lancashire and South Cumbria. Offering free professional therapy services delivered by qualified and highly experienced staff, including counselling, hypnotherapy, The Alexander Technique, aromatherapy massage, group activities and support groups. Has a child and young people's service.
Web: www.cancercare.org.uk
Lancaster Ph: 01524 381 820
Kendal Ph: 01539 7358009
Barrow Ph: 0129 836 926

Cancer Research UK

Working to bring forward the day when all cancers are cured. Funding research and developing policy to accelerate progress and reach the goal of 75% survival within the next 20 years.
Web: www.cancerresearchuk.org
Ph: 0300 123 1022

Cancer Support Centre Weston Park

Supporting anyone affected by cancer through a range of services run by healthcare professionals.
Web: www.cancersupportcentre.co.uk
Ph: 0114 226 5666

Cancer Support UK

Providing practical and emotional support to people with cancer, during and after treatment.
Web: www.cancersupportuk.org
Ph: 020 7470 8755

Cancer Support Yorkshire

Offering practical and emotional support to people affected by a cancer diagnosis. Providing assistance with transport, welfare rights and finances, counselling, complementary therapies and a range of classes and groups.
Web: www.cancersupportyorkshire.org.uk
Ph: 01274 77 66 88

Chai Cancer Support

Comprehensive, professional and expert services for any member of the Jewish community affected by cancer. There are eight centre nationally in North West London, South London, Redbridge, Hackney, Southend, Leeds, North Manchester, Liverpool, South Manchester and Glasgow.
Web: www.chaicancercare.org
Ph: 0208 202 2211
Helpline Ph: 00808 808 4567

Children with Cancer UK

A mission to improve survival rates and the quality of survival in young cancer patients. Funding research to find ways to prevent cancer in the future.
Web: www.childrenwithcancer.org.uk
Ph: 020 7404 0808

CLAN Cancer Support

Support services for those affected by cancer across north-east Scotland, Orkney and Shetland. 10 wellbeing centres to help people live with and beyond their or their loved ones cancer diagnosis.
Web: www.clanhouse.org
Ph: 01224 647 000

The Clatterbridge Cancer Charity

Transforming cancer care for patients and research at The Clatterbridge Cancer Centre.
Web: www.clatterbridgecc.nhs.uk
Ph: 0151 556 5566

CLIC Sargent

Helping young people and their families with day-to-day support, financial assistance, home nurse care and CLIC Sargent accommodation located close to hospitals to keep families together during treatment.
Web: www.clicsargent.org.uk
Ph: 0300 330 0803

Dimbleby Cancer Care

Offers care and support to people and their families who are living with cancer.
Web: www.dimblebycancercare.org
Ph: 020 7188 7889

DKMS

Deleting blood cancer by recruiting and retaining potential blood cell donors to give a second chance of life to people with blood cancer.
Web: www.dkms.org.uk
Ph: 020 8747 5620

EHE Rare Cancer Charity

Epithelioid Haemangioendothelioa (EHE) is a rare form of cancer. This organisation is working to gather data worldwide with sister branches in the US and Australia to further research and to support patients with this disease.
Web: www.ehercc.org.uk

The Eve Appeal

The only UK national charity raising awareness and funding research into the five gynaecological cancers – womb, ovarian, vulval and vaginal.
Web: www.eveappeal.org.uk
Ph: 020 7605 0108

Eyes on the Prize

Information and support for HPV Oropharyngeal Cancer patients.
Web: www.eyesontheprize.info

F

C

K

Fight Bladder Cancer UK

Run by bladder cancer survivors and their families to support everyone affected by bladder cancer. Raising awareness and aiming to achieve better outcomes and quality of life for all those affected.
Web: www.fightbladdercancer.co.uk

Future Dreams

Support, awareness and research for those touched by breast cancer. Providing emotional and physical support and therapies for women and their families.
Web: www.futuredreams.org.uk
Ph: 0808 800 6000

G

GIST Support UK

Support and information for patients and carers with gastro-intestinal stomal tumours.
Web: www.gistsupportuk.com

H

Heartburn Cancer UK

Providing support for sufferers of oesophageal cancer, particularly those diagnosed with Barrett's. Raising awareness about checking symptoms of persistent heartburn as a warning sign of this disease.
Web: www.heartburncanceruk.org
Ph: 01256 338 668

I

The Institute of Cancer Research

One of the world's most influential cancer research organisations.
Web: www.icr.ac.uk
Ph: 020 7352 8133

The International Brain Tumour Alliance

A unique global network for brain tumour patient and carer groups around the world.
Web: www.theibta.org
Ph: 1737 813 872

U
K

It's In The Bag

New diagnoses information, survivorship toolkits and personal development weekends for men with testicular cancer in the South-West of England.
Web: www.itsinthebag.org.uk
Ph: 075 060 13762

It's On The Ball

Awareness talks, buddy support system for newly diagnosed testicular cancer patients.
Web: www.itsontheball.org
Ph: 073 757 95453

J

Jo's Cervical Cancer Trust

For women, their families and friends affected by cervical cancer and cervical abnormalities. Providing quality information and support. Campaigning for excellence in cervical cancer treatment and prevention.
Web: www.jostrust.org.uk
Ph: 0800 802 8000

K

Kidney Cancer Association UK

A charitable organisation comprising patients, family members, physicians, researchers and other health professionals globally. Dedicated to the eradication of death and suffering from renal cancers.
Web: www.kidneycancer.org
Ph: 020 3432 6491

Kidney Cancer UK

Provides the UK's first free, dedicated Kidney Cancer Counselling Service. Information on clinical trials, resource information and support for patients.
Web: www.kcuk.org.uk
Ph: 01223 870008

Kidscan

Dedicated to beating childhood cancer. Working to ensure that every child diagnosed with cancer can survive and thrive through to adulthood.
Web: www.kidscan.org.uk
Ph: 0161 295 3864

Kids Cancer Charity

A national charity set up to support children with cancer and their families. Offering family services, holiday and staycations.
Web: www.kidscancercharity.org
Ph: 01792 480 500

Leighton Linslade Cancer Support Group

Support for anyone affected by cancer. Located in Bedfordshire.
Web: www.e-voice.org.uk
Ph: 01525 851 932

Leukaemia Care

A national blood cancer charity that provides emotional support, advice and help to anyone affected by blood cancer.
Web: www.leukaemiacare.org.uk
Ph: 0808 801 0444

Look Good Feel Better

Offers free skincare and make-up workshops to create a sense of support and wellbeing for women struggling with the side-effects of cancer treatment.
Web: www.lookgoodfeelbetter.co.uk

Lymphoedema Support Network

Award winning charity providing information and support for those living with or affected by lymphoedema and chronic oedema.
Web: www.lymphoedema.org
Ph: 020 7351 44 80

Lymphoma Action

Information, support and connection to other patients with lymphoma. Support groups, buddy support, online forums and helpline all dedicated exclusively to lymphoma.
Web: www.lymphoma-action.org.uk
Ph: 0808 808 5555

M
U
K

Macmillan Cancer Support

Macmillan is an incredible resource comprised of cancer patients, survivors, supporters, professionals, volunteers and campaigners providing support, information and inspiration for your entire cancer journey.
Web: www.macmillan.org.uk
Ph: 0800 808 00 00

Maggie's Centres

Centres that help anyone affected by cancer. Their 21 centres are staffed by cancer support specialists, advisors, nutritionists, therapists and psychologists to provide support that best suits you.
Web: www.maggiescentre.org
Ph: 0300 123 1801

Marie Curie

Giving care and support to people living with any terminal illness and their families.
Web: www.mariecure.org.uk
Ph: 0800 716 146

Melanoma UK

Personal support, guidance and treatment for those affected by melanoma.
Web: www.melanomauk.org.uk
Ph: 0808 171 2455

Mouth Cancer Foundation

Information and access to support groups for people suffering from mouth cancer.
Web: www.mouthcancerfoundation.org
Ph: 020 8940 2222

Myeloma UK

Help and support, resources and information for patients, carers and family members affected by myeloma.
Web: www.myeloma.org.uk
Ph: 0131 557 3332

NET Patient Foundation

Support services and access to support groups for those affected by Neuroendocrine tumours.

Web:www.netpatientfoundation.org

Ph: 01926 883 487

The Nightingale Cancer Support Centre

Helping people affected by cancer by developing a tailor-made programme for each person.

Web: www.nightingalesupport.org.uk

Ph: 020 8366 4333

Noah's Ark Children's Hospital Charity

Supporting the Noah's Ark Children's Hospital for Wales in providing world class care, helping to ensure the best outcome and experience possible for children and their families.

Web: www.noahsarkcharity.org

Ph: 029 2184 7310

OcuMel UK

A site run by eye cancer patients and their family members. Providing information to those affected by eye cancer.

Web: www.ocumeluk.org

Ph: 0300 790 0512

Oesophageal Patients Association

Helping patients, carers and their families to cope with oesophageal and gastric cancer.

Web: www.opa.org.uk

Ph: 0121 704 9860

Orchid

An organisation focused on fighting male cancer including testicular, prostate and penile cancers through pioneering research and promoting awareness.

Web: www.orchid-cancer.org.uk

Ph: 0800 802 0010

Ovacome

Providing a strong, supportive and knowledgeable community for anyone affected by ovarian cancer.
Web: www.ovacome.org.uk
Ph: 0800 008 7054

Ovarian Cancer Action

Information and resources for those diagnosed with ovarian cancer. Involved with funding research, raising awareness and campaigning for change to prevent hereditary ovarian cancer.
Web: www.ovarian.org.uk
Ph: 020 7380 2730

Pancreatic Cancer UK

Information about pancreatic cancer including diagnosis, treatment options, managing symptoms and living with pancreatic cancer. Specialist nurse available on helpline.
Web: www.pancreaticcancer.org.uk
Ph: 0800 801 0707

Paul's Cancer Support Centre

Helping people affected by cancer, their families and anyone who supports them, in Battersea and through a Home Vising Service.
Web: www.paulsancersupportcentre.org.uk
Ph: 020 7924 3924

PCaSO Prostate Cancer Support Organisation

A charity for men diagnosed with prostate cancer, run by patients diagnosed with prostate cancer.
Web: www.pcasoprostatecancersouth.org
Ph: 0800 035 5302

Prevent Breast Cancer

The only UK breast cancer charity funding ground-breaking research solely aimed at preventing the disease for future generations.
Web: www.preventbreastcancer.org.uk
Ph: 0161 291 4400

Prostate Cancer UK

Shifting the science to focus on radical improvements in diagnosis, treatment, prevention and support to stop men dying from prostate cancer.

Web: www.prostatecanceruk.org

Ph: 0800 082 1616

Pseudomyxoma Survivor

Providing support to people affected by pseudomyxoma peritonei, appendix cancer and other peritoneal surface malignancy in the form of emotional support and practical advice through an online community. Offers support to patients all over the world.

Web: www.pseudomyxomasurvivor.org

Ph: 300 30 200 50

Riprap

A site developed especially for teenagers who have a parent with cancer. Answers questions and connects teenagers to others going through the same experiences.

Web: www.riprap.org.uk

The Robin Cancer Trust

A germ cell cancer awareness charity. Raising awareness about testicular and ovarian cancer.

Web: www.therobincancertrust.org

Ph: 07874 069 778

Roy Castle Lung Cancer Foundation

Resources and information for those dealing with lung cancer.

Web: www.roycastle.org

Ph: 0333 323 7200

S

U

K

Shine Cancer Support

Supporting adults in their 20s, 30s, and 40s who have experienced a cancer diagnosis. Tailors information and peer support in a way that suits the lifestyle of this age group with activities such as lunches and drinks evening, beach walks, getaways, networking and mentoring.
Web: www.shinecancersupport.org

SimPal

Aiming to make change within the cancer sector and to support as many people as possible who are living with cancer by providing free mobile communication.
Web: www.yoursimpal.com
Ph: 0800 567 7890

Skcin

The Karen Clifford Skin Cancer Charity is intent on raising awareness of skin cancer through education, promoting prevention and early detection. Information downloads and resources.
Web: www.skcin.org
Ph: 0115 9819 116

Starlight Children's Foundation

A national children's charity that is dedicated to brightening the lives of children and teenager suffering from a serious or terminal illness.
Web: www.starlight.org.uk
Ph: 020 7262 2881

T

Tackle Prostate Cancer

Acting as the voice of prostate cancer patients and their families. Encouraging and assisting the formation and development of patient-led support groups throughout the UK.
Web: www.tackprostate.org
Ph: 0800 035 5302

Target Ovarian Cancer

The UK's leading ovarian cancer charity. Working to improve early detection, fund life-saving research and to provide much-needed support to women with ovarian cancer.
Web: www.targetovariancancer.org.uk
Ph: 020 7923 5470

Teenage Cancer Trust

Providing life-changing care for young people aged between 13 and 24. They bring young people together to be treated by teenage cancer experts and run age relevant events and workshops.
Web: www.teenagecancertrust.org
Ph: 020 7612 0370

Tenovus Cancer Care

Delivering cancer treatment, emotional support and practical advice to the heart of the community with mobile support units and a support line manned by qualified nurses.
Web: www.tenovuscancercare.org.uk
Ph: 0800 808 1010

Testicular Cancer Network US

A consortium of testicular cancer awareness, support and research charities working together to save the lives of men across the UK.
Web: www.testicularcancernetwork.co.uk

Throat Cancer Foundation

Raising awareness of cancers affect the head, mouth and neck. Information and resources.
Web: www.throatcancerfoundation.org
Ph: 0203 4754 065

Topic of Cancer

Funding research for immunotherapy treatments. Local support groups provide support and activities for patients, survivors, carers and families.
Web: www.topciofcancer.org.uk
Ph: 01372 456 025

U

UK and Bradford Cancer Support
A resource for cancer patients diagnosed with cancer.
Web: www.bradfordcancersupport.org.uk

W

Wendy Gough Cancer Awareness Foundation
Raising awareness of testicular and breast cancer in schools, clubs and workplaces.
Web: www.wgcaf.com

White House Cancer Support
A volunteer organisation providing support for people affected by cancer across the Black Country. Offering help with transport, complementary therapies, support groups and care.
Web: www.support4cancer.org.uk
Ph: 01384 231 232

Womb Cancer Support UK
A national voluntary organisation offering support to women who have been diagnosed with womb cancer.
Web: www.wombcancersupportuk.weebly.com

Y

U
X

York Against Cancer
A local charity helping patients and their families in York and North Yorkshire.
Web: www.yorkagainstcancer.org.uk
Ph: 01904 764 466

YouCan
Wellbeing services to support young people up to the age of 35 impacted by cancer. Funding short breaks by the Kent seaside.
Web: www.youcan.org.uk
Ph: 01732 844 874

The Youth Cancer Trust
Organises free, activity-based holidays for young people with cancer aged 14 to 30 who have been patients of any UK hospital. Also available to those in remission for up to five years or those living with the late effects of having had cancer as a teenager.
Web: www.youthcancertrust.org
Ph: 01202 763 591

USA

A

U
S
A

Abramson Cancer Center

A world leader in cancer research, patient care and education. Offering cancer patients with the newest and most innovative therapeutic advances.
Web: www.pennmedicine.org
Ph: 800 789 7366

Adrenal Cancer Support

Information gathered from Adrenal Cancer patients.
Web: www.adrenocorticalcarcinoma.org

Aim At Melanoma

Globally engaged and locally invested in advancing the battle against melanoma through innovative research, legislative reform, education and patient and caregiver support.
Web: www.aimatmelanoma.org

Alex's Lemonade Stand Foundation

Changing the lives of children with cancer by funding impactful research, raising awareness, supporting families and empowering everyone to help cure childhood cancer.
Web: www.alexslemonade.org
Ph: 866 333 1213

Alliance for Childhood Cancer

Provides a forum of national patient advocacy groups and medical scientific organisations that meet to share ideas, concerns and to work collaboratively to advance research and policies to prevent cancer, improve public education, diagnosis, treatment and the supportive care and survivorship of children and adolescents with cancer.
Web: www.allianceforchildhoolcancer.org

American Bladder Cancer Society

Functions to raise awareness of bladder cancer and to advocate for the advancement of research into a cure, treatment, early diagnosis and quality of life issues of survivors.
Web: www.bladdercancersupport.org

U S A

American Brain Tumor Association
Dedicated to brain tumour education, support and research. An advocate on behalf of the brain tumour community. Helping patients, caregivers and their loved ones to navigate the brain tumour journey.
Web: www.abta.org
Ph: 773 577 8750

American Cancer Society
Funds and conducts research, sharing expert information, supporting patients, and spreading the word about prevention.
Web: www.cancer.org
Ph: 800 227 2345

American Childhood Cancer Organization
Formed by a group of parents whose children were diagnosed with cancer, this organisation is committed to making the lives of children and families suffering from this disease and its long-term side-effects, easier.
Web: www.acco.org
Ph: 855 858 2226

American Lung Association
Working to save lives by improving lung health and preventing lung disease through education, advocacy and research.
Web: www.lung.org
Ph: 1 800 586 4872

Bandaides & Blackboards
A site helping people understand what it's like to grow up with medical problems, from the perspective of the children and teens who are doing just that.
Web: www.lehman.cuny.edu/faculty/jfleitas/bandaides/

Bladder Cancer Advocacy Network
Devoted to advancing bladder cancer research and supporting those impacted by the disease.
Web: www.bcan.org
Ph: 301 215 9099

U S A

Bladder Cancer

On the front-lines advocating for greater public awareness and increasing funding for research. Helping thousands of patients, caregivers and the medical community with educational resources and support services as they navigate their bladder cancer journey.
Web: www.bcan.org
Ph: 888 901 2226

Bladder Cancer Café

Treatment information, support and resources. Offers answers to relieve some of the fear and to reinforce hope to help patients and loved ones to find the best path.
Web: www.blcwebcafe.org

Blue Faery – The Adrienne Wilson Liver Cancer Association

Working to prevent, treat and cure primary liver cancer and to improve the quality of life for patients and caregivers with hope, information, and a voice.
Web: www.bluefaery.org
Ph: 818 636 5624

Breastcancer.org

Helping women, men and their loved ones make sense of the complex medical and personal information about breast health and breast cancer.
Web: www.breastancer.org
Ph: 610 642 6550

Breast Cancer Support

A site for breast cancer survivors to find support, information and to connect to someone who has experienced a similar diagnosis.
Web: www.bcsupport.org

BreastFree

Information, advice and support for women considering breast reconstruction.
Web: www.breastfree.org

Bright Pink

Putting breast and ovarian health awareness in action. Education, information and support for people with these cancers.

Web: www.brightpink.org

Camp Mak-A-Dream

Empowering survivors and their families to live with and beyond cancer through life-changing experiences where they strengthen life skills, gain resilience and develop lasting relationships.

Web: www.campdream.org

Cancer.com

Providing clarity in the search for cancer resources. A curated selection of information from respected sources.

Web: www.cancer.com

Ph: 1 800 526 7736

Cancer.net

Trusted, compassionate information for people with cancer and their families and caregivers from the American Society of Clinical Oncology, the voice of the world's cancer physicians and oncology professionals.

Web: www.cancer.net

Ph: 571 483 1780

Ph: 888 651 3038

Cancercare

An organisation that offers counselling, support, education and financial assistance for patients, survivors, caregivers and loved ones.

Web: www.cancercare.org

Ph: 800 813 4673

Cancer Compass

A place to discover and share cancer-related information with people affected by cancer. Join to read message boards and join discussion forums.

Web: www.cancercompass.com

Cancer Hope Network

Offering on-on-one peer support for adults impacted by cancer.
Web: www.canerhopenetwork.org
Ph: 877 4673 638

Cancer Support Community

Extensive resources and information to access cancer support
throughout the USA.
Web: www.cancersupportcommunity.org
Ph: 888 793 9355

Chai Lifeline

Provides activities and events, Camp Simcha experiences, counselling,
crisis intervention and support for families with children who are
seriously ill.
Web: www.chailifeline.org
Ph: 212 465 1300

Caring Bridge

A place to create free, personal and private websites to connect family
and friends during a health challenge.
Web: www.caringbridge.org
Ph: 651 789 2300

Center for Cancer Research

A place to find information on clinical trials and research.
Web: www.ccr.cancer.gov

Chemocare

Information on your chemotherapy drugs and on managing side-effects.
Web: www.chemocare.com
Ph: 844 268 3901
Ph: 416 489 6440

Children's Cause Cancer Advocacy

The leading national advocacy organisation working to achieve access to less toxic and more effective paediatric cancer therapies; to expand resources for research and specialised care; and to address the unique needs and challenges of childhood cancer survivors and their families.
Web: www.childrenscause.org
Ph: 202 552 7392

Clinical Trials

A database of over 280,000 research studies in 204 countries. A great place to search for actively recruiting studies that you may be able to participate in or learn about new interventions/treatments that are being considered.
Web: www.clinicaltrials.gov

City of Hope Cancer Center

Pioneers at the forefront of cancer treatments. Offers clinical trials and comprehensive assistance for patients and their families through education, support groups, social resources and mind-body therapies.
Web: www.cityofhope.org
Ph: 800 826 4673

Coalition Against Childhood Cancer

Putting children and their families first to actively fight childhood cancer.
Web: www.ca2.org

Colorectal Cancer Alliance

Provides genuine support for patients, families, caregivers and survivors. Raising awareness of preventative measures and inspiring efforts to fund critical research.
Web: www.ccalliance.org
Ph: 877 422 2030

Corporate Angel Network

Has the sole mission of transporting cancer patients to hospitals for specialised treatment.
Web: www.corangelnetwork.org
Ph: 914 328 1313

Cure Search for Children's Cancer

Accelerating the search for cures for childhood cancers by driving innovation, overcoming research barriers and solving the field's most challenging problems. Provides resources and education.
Web: www.curesearch.org
Ph: 800 458 6223

D

Daily Strength

A website connecting you to support groups of specific types of cancer. Access support groups on colon, breast, thyroid, ovarian oesophageal, renal, skin, lung, cervical, brain, pancreatic, liver, prostate, vulvar, uterine, myelodysplasia, head and neck, bladder, bone, gastric, carcinoid syndrome, mesothelioma, rhabdomyosarcoma, vaginal cancer.
Web: https://www.dailystrength.org/categories/Cancers

Dana-Farber Cancer Institute

With a sole mission of defeating cancer, this Institute has been making life-changing breakthroughs in cancer research and patient care for over 70 years. They provide an individual treatment plan, integrative therapies counselling, plus patient and family support services.
Web: www.dana-farber.org
Ph: 617 632 3000

Debbie's Dream

A non-profit with the ultimate goal of making a cure for stomach cancer a reality. Raising awareness, advancing funding for research and providing education and support internationally to patients, families and caregivers.
Web: www.debbiesdream.org
Ph: 855 475 1200
Ph: 954 475 1200

E

Emerging Med

A site to help identify available clinical trials that match a specific diagnosis and treatment.
Web: www.emergingmed.com

F

U

S

A

Facing Our Risk of Cancer Empowered

FORCE improves the lives of individuals and families affected by hereditary breast, ovarian and related cancers.
Web: www.facingourrisk.org
Ph: 866 288 7475

Family Caregiver Alliance

An online service for quality information, support and resources for caregivers.
Web: www.caregiver.org
Ph: 800 445 8106
Ph: 415 434 3388

Foundation for Women's Cancer

Has a vision to eradicate gynaecologic cancers. Supports research, education and public awareness of gynaecologic cancers.
Web: www.foundationforwomenscancer.org
Ph: 312 578 1439

Fight Colorectal Cancer

A community of patients, fighters and champions pushing for better policies and to support research, education and awareness for all those touched by colorectal cancer.
Web: www.fightcolorectalcancer.org
Ph: 703 548 1225

4th Angel

A patient and caregiver mentoring program. Free, one-on-one confidential outreach and support from someone who has successfully made the same journey.
Web: www.4thangel.org

Friends of Scott (Friends to Children with Cancer)

Founded in memory of Scott Delgadillo who lost his life to childhood cancer. Providing emotional and financial support needed to cope with this disease.
Web: www.friendsofscott.org

Global Initiative Against HPV and Cervical Cancer

Working with programs domestically within the US and internationally to promote health education, train and engage communities in HPV vaccination, screening and early treatment programs.

Web: www.giahc.org

Ph: 800 552 4375

Head & Neck Cancer Guide

Information and support for patients and caregivers on diagnosis, treatment and dealing with emotions for people impacted by Head and Neck Cancer.

Web: www.headandneckcancerguide.org

HER2 Support

A support group comprising patients, caregivers, mothers, daughters, sons and husbands of breast cancer survivors who are HER2 positive.

Web: www.her2support.org

His Prostate Cancer

For patients, loved ones and caregivers who have been affected by prostate cancer. Get information and support to help deal with the effects of prostate cancer.

Web: www.hisprostatecancer.com

HysterSisters

Personalised support and information dedicated to the medical and emotional issues surrounding the hysterectomy experience, a procedure that often accompanies women with gynaecologic cancers. A woman-to-woman source of information.

Web: www.hystersisters.com

I

U S A

Imaginary Friend Society
A site with kid-friendly videos covering a wide range of cancer-related topics, everything from defining cancer itself to chemotherapy and MRIs.
Web: www.imaginaryfriendsociety.com

Imerman Angels
Provides personalised connections that enable one-on-one support among cancer fighters, survivors and caregivers.
Web: www.imermanangels.org
Ph: 866 463 7626

Inflammatory Breast Cancer Research Foundation
Improving the lives of those touched by inflammatory breast cancer through the power of action and advocacy.
Web: www.ibcresearch.org

Intercultural Cancer Council
Working to eliminate the unequal burden of cancer among racial and ethnic minorities and medically undeserved populations in the United States and its associated territories.
Web: www.interculturalcancercouncil.org

International Myeloma Foundation
Improving the quality of life of more than 500,000 myeloma patient members in 140 countries.
Web: www.myeloma.org
Ph: 800 452 2873
Ph: 818 487 7455

International Neuroendocrine Cancer Alliance
The global advocate for neuroendocrine cancer patients. Working to ensure all neuroendocrine cancer patients get a timely diagnosis, the best care and ultimately, a cure. Branches in countries all around the world.
Web: www.incalliance.org

J

John Hopkins Medicine: The Sidney Kimmel Comprehensive Cancer Center

Recognised by the National Cancer Institute as a "Center of Excellence", this centre is a leader in research and provides a full range of preventative, diagnostic, therapeutic, supportive and patient focussed services to cancer patients and their families.
Web: www.hopkinsmedicine.org/kimmel_cancer_center/
Ph: 410 955 5000

K

Kidney Cancer Association

A charitable organisation comprising patients, family members, physicians, researchers and other health professionals globally. It is the world's first international charity dedicated specifically to the eradication of death and suffering from renal cancers.
Web: www.kidneycancer.org
Ph: 800 850 9132

L

USA

Leukaemia and Lymphoma Society

Has a mission to cure leukaemia, lymphoma, Hodgkin's disease and myeloma and to improve the quality of life of patients and their families.
Web: www.lls.orgPh: 888 557 7177

LIVESTRONG

Aims to improve the lives of people affected by cancer by providing direct services, providing resources and connecting people and communities with the services they need.
Web: www.livestrong.org
Ph: 855 220 7777

Living Beyond Breast Cancer

Providing programs and services to help people whose lives have been impacted by breast cancer. Offering information, community and resources reviewed by some of the country's leading healthcare experts.
Web: www.ibbc.org
Ph: 855 807 6386
Ph: 610 645 4567

U S A

Look Good Feel Better

Teaching cancer patients how to manage the appearance-related side-effects caused by cancer treatment. Women, men and teens participate in a practical workshop which covers skincare, make-up and headwear demonstrations leaving them empowered and ready to face their cancer diagnosis with confidence.
Web: www.lookgoodfeelbetter.org

Lungcancer.org

Providing free, professional support including counselling, support groups, financial assistance, educational workshops and publications to anyone coping with lung cancer.
Web: www.lungcancer.org
Ph: 800 813 4673

Lung Cancer Alliance

Supporting you through every stage of lung cancer. Information, one-on-one help and support.
Web: www.lungcanceralliance.org
Ph: 1800 298 2436

Lung Cancer Research Foundation

Improving lung cancer outcomes by funding research for the prevention, diagnosis, treatment and cure of lung cancer.
Web: www.lungcancerresearchfoundation.org
Ph: 212 588 1580

LUNGevity Foundation

Changing outcomes for people with lung cancer through research, education and support.
Web: www.lungevity.org
Ph: 844 360 5864

Lymphoma Coalition

A worldwide network of lymphoma patient groups to create a level playing field of information around the world and to facilitate a community of lymphoma patient organisations to support one another's efforts in helping patients with lymphoma receive the care and support needed.
Web: www.lymphomacoalition.org

Lymphoma Research Foundation
Committed to eradicating lymphoma and serving those touched by this disease.
Web: www.lymphoma.org
Ph: 800 500 9976

Malecare
A website providing access to support groups for early stage, advanced stage and gay men's prostate cancer groups. Also has erectile dysfunction group and male breast cancer groups.
Web: www.malecare.org

Melanoma International Foundation
Created to provide scientifically sound guidance and support for melanoma patients. Their vision is to make top-notch melanoma treatment accessible to all patients globally.
Web: www.melanomainternational.org
Ph: 866 463 6663

Melanoma Research Foundation
Committed to the support of medical research in finding effective treatments and eventually a cure for melanoma. Also educates patients, caregivers and physicians about the prevention, diagnosis and treatment of melanoma.
Web: www.melanoma.org
Ph: 800 673 1290
Ph: 202 347 9678

The Mayo Clinic
For 150 years, Mayo Clinic has been known as the "hospital for hope when there is no hope." Ranked No. 1 Hospital by the U.S. News and World Report.
Web: www.mayoclinic.org
Ph: 480 301 8000

MD Anderson Center

Focussed exclusively on cancer. Ranked the no. 1 hospital for cancer care in the nation by U.S. News & World Report's "Best Hospitals" survey.
Web: www.mdanderson.org
Ph: 1 855 549 4047

Melanoma Research Foundation

Committed to supporting research and to educating and helping patients, caregivers and physicians about the prevention, diagnosis and treatment of melanoma. The oldest and largest online community of people affected by melanoma.
Web: www.melanoma.org
Ph: 800 673 1290

Memorial Sloan Kettering Cancer Center

Cancer care is the only thing they do. Their specialist treat every type of cancer with a philosophy of personalised care. They provide a treatment plan that fits your whole life. Staffed by world class surgeons, doctors and researchers, they turn today's scientific discoveries into tomorrow's treatments.
Web: www.mskcc.org
Ph: 212 639 2000

Men Against Breast Cancer

Providing targeted support services that educate and empower men to be effective caregivers when cancer strikes. A philosophy of leveraging the support of the whole family to help the patient with special emphasis on the important role of men in caring for the women they love.
Web: www.menagainstbreastcancer.org
Ph: 866 547 6222

The Metacancer Foundation

Resources and support for metastatic cancer survivors and their caregivers. Encourages dialogue among those with very different types of metastatic cancer as the psychological and emotional realities faced form a common bond.
Web: www.metacancer.org

Multiple Myeloma Foundation
A patient-founded and patient-focused site fighting for a world where every person has precisely what they need to prevent or defeat multiple myeloma.
Web: www.themmrf.org
Ph: 203 229 0464

Musella Foundation
Dedicated to helping brain tumour patients through emotional and financial support, education, advocacy and raising money for brain tumour research.
Web: www.virtualtrials.com
Ph: 516 295 2870

National Brain Tumor Society
Fiercely committed to finding better treatments and a cure for people living with a brain tumour today and anyone who will be diagnosed tomorrow.
Web: www.braintumor.org
Ph: 617 924 9997

National Breast Cancer Foundation
Aims to provide help and inspiration to those affected by breast cancer through early detection, education and support services.
Web: www.nationalbreastcancer.org

National Cancer information Center
Information and support for those facing cancer, 24 hours a day, 365 days a year. Talk to trained information specialists who can connect patients, family and caregivers to valuable services and resources in their community.
Ph: 1 800 227 2345

National Cancer Institute
The nation's leader in cancer research. The NCI leads, conducts and supports cancer research across the USA to advance scientific knowledge and help all people live longer, healthier lives.
Web: www.cancer.gov
Ph: 1800 422 6237

U S A

National Cervical Cancer Coalition
A grassroots organisation dedicated to serving women with, or at risk of cervical cancer and HPV disease. Merged with the American Sexual Health Association, a non-profit with a long history of educating and raising awareness on sexual health issues.
Web: www.nccc-online.org
Ph: 800 685 5531

The National Children's Cancer Society
Providers of financial and emotional support for families facing childhood cancer.
Web: www.thenccs.org
Ph: 314 241 1600

National Coalition For Cancer Survivorship
Advocating for quality cancer care for all individuals touched by cancer.
Web: www.canceradvocacy.org
Ph: 877 622 7937

National Lymphedema Network
Providing education and guidance on lymphedema management to patients, healthcare professionals and the general public by disseminating information on prevention and management of primary and secondary lymphedema.
Web: www.lymphnet.org
Ph: 800 541 3259

National Marrow Donor Program
The largest and most diverse marrow registry in the world. Working every day to save lives for the thousands of people diagnosed every year with life-threatening blood cancers like leukaemia and lymphoma.
Web: www.bethematch.org
Ph: 1800 627 7692

National Ovarian Cancer Coalition
Fighting tirelessly to prevent and cure ovarian cancer and to improve quality of life for survivors.
Web: www.ovarian.org
Ph: 888 682 7426
Ph: 214 273 4200

Native American Cancer Research
Dedicated to helping improve the lives of Native American cancer patients and survivors.
Web: www.natamcancer.org
Ph: 1 800 537 8295

No Stomach for Cancer
Supporting research and uniting the caring power of people worldwide affected by stomach cancer.
Web: www.nostomachforcancer.org
Ph: 608 692 5141

Nueva Vida
Informing, supporting and empowering Latinas whose lives are affected by cancer.
Web: www.nueva-vida.org
Baltimore Ph: 410 916 2150
DC Ph: 202 223 9100

Ocular Melanoma Foundation
To accelerate and enhance scientific research, advocacy and awareness of ocular melanoma and to provide education and support to patients, their families and healthcare professionals.
Web: www.ocularmelanoma.org
Ph: 202 684 9380

Oncolink
Resources and links to information and support services for all types of cancer.
Web: www.oncolink.org

The Oral Cancer Foundation
Provides direct peer-to-peer support for oral cancer patients and their caregivers.
Web: www.oralcancerfoundation.org
Ph: 949 723 4400

Ovarian Cancer Research Alliance

A mission to cure ovarian cancer, advocate for patients and support survivors.

Web: www.ocrahope.org

Ph: 212 268 1002

Pancreatic Cancer Action Network

Fighting pancreatic cancer on all fronts: research, clinical initiatives, patient services and advocacy.

Web: www.pancan.org

Ph: 877 573 9971

Pancreatica

A site serving as a worldwide gathering point for the latest news and information regarding clinical trials and other responsible medical care in the treatment of pancreatic cancer.

Web: www.pancreatica.org

Ph: 831 658 0600

Patient Advocate Foundation

A national non-profit organisation which provides case management services and financial aid to Americans.

Web: www.patientadvocate.org

Ph: 800 532 5274

People Against Childhood Cancer

An advocacy community on a mission to raise awareness of childhood cancer. A great resource to find local support.

Web: www.curechildhoodcancer.ning.com

Phoenix5

Helping men and their companions overcome the effects of prostate cancer.

Web: www.phoenix5.org

Prevent Cancer Foundation

Committed to stop cancer before it starts through research, education, outreach and advocacy.

Web: www.preventcancer.org

Ph: 800 227 2732

Ph: 703 836 4412

Prostate Cancer Foundation

Funding the world's most promising research to improve prevention, detection and treatment of prostate cancer.

Web: www.pcf.org

Ph: 1 800 757 2873

Ph: 310 570 4700

The Roslyn Carter Institute for Caregiving

Establishes local, state, national and international partnerships committed to building quality, long-term, home and community-based services. Offering advocacy, education, research and support for caregivers.

Web: www.rosalynncarter.org

Ph: 229 928 1234

Save My Fertility

An authoritative resource for cancer patients who want to learn more about preserving their fertility before and during cancer treatment and protecting their hormonal health after treatment.

Web: www.savemyfertility.org

Ph: 312 503 2504

Share Cancer Support

Creating and sustaining a supportive community of women affected by breast or ovarian cancer.

Web: www.sharecancersupport.org

Ph: 844 275 7427

Ph: 212 719 0364

Sisters Network

Committed to creating local and national attention about the devastating impact that breast cancer has in the Africa American community.
Web: www.sistersnetworkinc.org
Ph: 713 781 0255

Skin Cancer Foundation

On a mission to save lives by educating the community about skin cancer.
Web: www.skincancer.org
Ph: 212 725 5176

Spinal Cord Tumor Association

Seeks to support spinal cord tumour survivors and their families and to educate and raise awareness about this rare and debilitating illness.
Web: www.spinalcordtumor.org

St Baldrick's Foundation

Funding research to more than 373 institutions treating kids with cancer in the US and around the world.
Web: www.stbaldricks.org
Ph: 888 899 2253

Starlight Children's Foundation US

Creating moments of joy and comfort to hospitalised children and their families. For 35 years, Starlight has brought smiles to more than 60 million critically, chronically and terminally ill children in the United States, Canada, Australia and the United Kingdom.
Web: www.starlight.org

Step Up, Speak Out

Resources, support and advocacy for women and men with breast cancer related lymphedema.
Web: www.stepup-speakout.org

Stupid Cancer

A leader in young adult cancer advocacy, research and support. "We connect you with your community and strive to make it all suck a little less." Their mission is to empower, support and improve health outcomes for the young adult cancer community.
Web: www.stupidcancer.org

Support for People with Oral and Head and Neck Cancer

Dedicated to raising awareness and meeting the needs of oral and head and neck cancer patients.
Web: www.spohnc.org
Ph: 1800 377 0928

Survivorship A to Z

Information and tools to empower you to live successfully with a cancer.
Web: www.survivorshipatoz.org

Susan G Komen

Saving lives by ensuring that all people receive the care they need. Finding breakthroughs to prevent and cure breast cancer.
Web: www.komen.org
Ph: 1 877 465 6636

TC Cancer.com

A site developed for the sole purpose of education and support for patients with testicular cancer and their family members. A resource network with a focus on connecting patients to support forums.
Web: www.tc-cancer.com

Testicular Cancer Awareness Foundation

Strives to spread awareness and support in the fight against testicular cancer.
Web: www.testicluarcancerawarenessfoundation.org

The Testicular Cancer resource Centre

Providing testicular cancer information and support.
Web: www.thetcrc.org

T.H.E. Brain Trust
Has the primary purpose of providing support to people affected by brain tumours and related conditions by hosting a diverse collection of online support groups.
Web: www.braintrust.org

13Thirty
Internationally known and respected in the field of adolescent and young adult cancer. Efforts are concentrated on providing resources, advocacy and support to help adolescents and young adults impacted by cancer to live their very best lives today.
Web:www.13thirty.org
Ph: 585 563 6221

ThyCa: Thyroid Cancer Survivors' Association
Created by thyroid cancer survivors to educate patients and families, communicate with health care professionals and to support research for a future free of thyroid cancer.
Web: www.thyca.org
Ph: 877 588 7904

Triple Negative Breast Cancer Foundation
A source of information for triple negative breast cancer patients, a catalyst for science and patient advocacy groups and a caring community with meaningful services for patients and their families.
Web: www.tnbcfoundation.org

The Ulman Cancer Fund for Young Adults
Changing lives by creating a community of support for young adults and their loved ones, impacted by cancer.
Web: www.ulmanfund.org
Ph: 410 964 0202

Us Too

Founded and governed by people affected directly by prostate cancer. A resource of volunteers with peer-to-peer support and educational materials to help men and their families and caregivers to make informed decisions about prostate cancer detection, treatment options and related side-effects.

Web: www.ustoo.org

Ph: 800 808 7866

Ph: 630 795 1002

Young Survival Coalition

Offers resources, connections and outreach for young women who are diagnosed with breast cancer.

Web: www.youngsurvival.org

Ph: 877 972 1011

Zero

Working to end prostate cancer. Information, education and support for patients, families and caregivers.

Web: www.zerocancer.org

Ph: 202 463 9455

SURVIVE & THRIVE

My Cancer Journey

WORKBOOK

My GP

Name _____

Address _____

Phone _____

Fax _____

Email _____

My Specialist Doctor

Name _____

Address _____

Phone _____

Fax _____

Email _____

My Specialist Doctor

Name _____

Address _____

Phone _____

Fax _____

Email _____

My Specialist Doctor

Name _____

Address _____

Phone _____

Fax _____

Email _____

My Diagnosis and Treatment Recommendations

Doctor/s _____

Diagnosis _____

_____

_____

Treatment _____

_____

_____

_____

_____

_____

_____

Questions for my Doctor/s

Question _____

Answer _____

_____

Question _____

Answer _____

_____

Question _____

Answer _____

_____

Question _____

Answer _____

_____

My Medical History

A comprehensive medical history provides your medical team with a full picture of your overall health. Knowledge will enable them to give you the most accurate diagnosis and the best possible treatment recommendation. Carefully fill out the sections below, including all of your past illnesses, surgery, treatments and medical procedures.

Date _____ **Doctor** _____

Notes _____

_____

_____

Date _____ **Doctor** _____

Notes _____

_____

_____

Date _____ **Doctor** _____

Notes _____

_____

_____

Date _____ **Doctor** _____

Notes _____

_____

_____

Date _____ **Doctor** _____

Notes _____

_____

_____

Date _____ **Doctor** _____

Notes _____

_____

_____

Date _____ **Doctor** _____

Notes _____

_____

_____

Date _____ **Doctor** _____

Notes _____

_____

_____

Date _____ **Doctor** _____

Notes _____

_____

_____

Date _____ **Doctor** _____

Notes _____

_____

_____

Date _____ **Doctor** _____

Notes _____

_____

_____

My Test Results

Correct diagnosis usually requires a variety of tests including CT Scans, biopsies, ultrasounds and more. As your treatment progresses, you will take more tests to assess your status. Track your progress by recording test results here.

Date _____ **Test** _____
Notes _____
_____
_____

Date _____ **Test** _____
Notes _____
_____
_____

Date _____ **Test** _____
Notes _____
_____
_____

Date _____ **Test** _____
Notes _____
_____
_____

Date _____ **Test** _____
Notes _____
_____
_____

Date _____ **Test** _____

Notes _____

_____

_____

_____

Date _____ **Test** _____

Notes _____

_____

_____

_____

Date _____ **Test** _____

Notes _____

_____

_____

_____

Date _____ **Test** _____

Notes _____

_____

_____

_____

Date _____ **Test** _____

Notes _____

_____

_____

_____

Date _____ **Test** _____

Notes _____

_____

_____

_____

Date _____ **Test** _____

Notes _____

_____

_____

Date _____ **Test** _____

Notes _____

_____

_____

Date _____ **Test** _____

Notes _____

_____

_____

Date _____ **Test** _____

Notes _____

_____

_____

Date _____ **Test** _____

Notes _____

_____

_____

Date _____ **Test** _____

Notes _____

_____

_____

_____

Date _____ **Test** _____
Notes _____
_____
_____

Date _____ **Test** _____
Notes _____
_____
_____

Date _____ **Test** _____
Notes _____
_____
_____

Date _____ **Test** _____
Notes _____
_____
_____

Date _____ **Test** _____
Notes _____
_____
_____

Date _____ **Test** _____
Notes _____
_____
_____

My Treatment Diary

This is the place to record each appointment you attend. Your primary support person can help you with this. By filling in these sections after each consultation you will have an accurate record to refer to when it is needed.

Date _____ **Doctor** _____
Notes _____
_____
_____

Date _____ **Doctor** _____
Notes _____
_____
_____

Date _____ **Doctor** _____
Notes _____
_____
_____

Date _____ **Doctor** _____
Notes _____
_____
_____

Date _____ **Doctor** _____
Notes _____
_____
_____
_____

Date _____ **Doctor** _____

Notes _____

_____

_____

Date _____ **Doctor** _____

Notes _____

_____

_____

Date _____ **Doctor** _____

Notes _____

_____

_____

Date _____ **Doctor** _____

Notes _____

_____

_____

Date _____ **Doctor** _____

Notes _____

_____

_____

Date _____ **Doctor** _____

Notes _____

_____

_____

Date _____ **Doctor** _____
Notes _____
_____
_____

Date _____ **Doctor** _____
Notes _____
_____
_____

Date _____ **Doctor** _____
Notes _____
_____
_____

Date _____ **Doctor** _____
Notes _____
_____
_____

Date _____ **Doctor** _____
Notes _____
_____
_____

Date _____ **Doctor** _____
Notes _____
_____
_____

Date _____ **Doctor** _____

Notes _____

_____

_____

Date _____ **Doctor** _____

Notes _____

_____

_____

Date _____ **Doctor** _____

Notes _____

_____

_____

Date _____ **Doctor** _____

Notes _____

_____

_____

Date _____ **Doctor** _____

Notes _____

_____

_____

Date _____ **Doctor** _____

Notes _____

_____

_____

_____

Date _____ **Doctor** _____

Notes _____

_____

_____

_____

Date _____ **Doctor** _____

Notes _____

_____

_____

_____

Date _____ **Doctor** _____

Notes _____

_____

_____

_____

Date _____ **Doctor** _____

Notes _____

_____

_____

_____

Date _____ **Doctor** _____

Notes _____

_____

_____

_____

Date _____ **Doctor** _____

Notes _____

_____

_____

_____

Date _____ **Doctor** _____

Notes _____

_____

_____

Date _____ **Doctor** _____

Notes _____

_____

_____

Date _____ **Doctor** _____

Notes _____

_____

_____

Date _____ **Doctor** _____

Notes _____

_____

_____

Date _____ **Doctor** _____

Notes _____

_____

_____

Date _____ **Doctor** _____

Notes _____

_____

_____

My Medication

It is imperative to keep accurate information on your medication, dosage and frequency. Fill in each section when a new medication is prescribed. Fill in the end date if the medication is discontinued. I have also included a chart so that if you have a number of medications, you can easily keep track.

Date _____ **Doctor** _____

Dosage _____ Frequency _____

_____

End Date (date medication discontinued) _____

Date _____ **Doctor** _____

Dosage _____ Frequency _____

_____

End Date (date medication discontinued) _____

Date _____ **Doctor** _____

Dosage _____ Frequency _____

_____

End Date (date medication discontinued) _____

Date _____ **Doctor** _____

Dosage _____ Frequency _____

_____

End Date (date medication discontinued) _____

Date _____ **Doctor** _____

Dosage _____ Frequency _____

_____

End Date (date medication discontinued) _____

Date ———— **Doctor** _____

Dosage ———— Frequency _____

_____

End Date (date medication discontinued) _____

Date ———— **Doctor** _____

Dosage ———— Frequency _____

_____

End Date (date medication discontinued) _____

Date ———— **Doctor** _____

Dosage ———— Frequency _____

_____

End Date (date medication discontinued) _____

Date ———— **Doctor** _____

Dosage ———— Frequency _____

_____

End Date (date medication discontinued) _____

Date ———— **Doctor** _____

Dosage ———— Frequency _____

_____

End Date (date medication discontinued) _____

Date ———— **Doctor** _____

Dosage ———— Frequency _____

_____

End Date (date medication discontinued) _____

Day	Medication	Dosage	AM	Noon	PM
Mon					
Tues					
Wed					
Thu					
Fri					
Sat					
Sun					

My Support Team

This is the place where your primary support person can record details of the people who have offered to help with meals, transport, financial assistance, home chores, babysitting etc. You can also record contacts at support organisations who have offered counselling and complementary therapy services. This ensures that if you as the patient is unwell, your support person will have all the contact information for the people who have offered help and can co-ordinate task directly with them. The list is also a way to ensure that you thank everyone for their support on your journey.

Name _____

Contact Number _____

Type of Assistance _____

Thanked _____

Name _____

Contact Number _____

Type of Assistance _____

Thanked _____

Name _____

Contact Number _____

Type of Assistance _____

Thanked _____

Name _____

Contact Number _____

Type of Assistance _____

Thanked _____

Name _____

Contact Number _____

Type of Assistance _____

Thanked _____

Name _____

Contact Number _____

Type of Assistance _____

Thanked _____

Name _____

Contact Number _____

Type of Assistance _____

Thanked _____

Name _____

Contact Number _____

Type of Assistance _____

Thanked _____

Name _____

Contact Number _____

Type of Assistance _____

Thanked _____

Name _____

Contact Number _____

Type of Assistance _____

Thanked _____

My Wellness Plan

You may choose to change your eating habit, to begin therapies or add supplements to your daily routine. Make a note of what you are doing so that you have a record for yourself and any medical professional who may need to know this information. Here is a checklist of things you may or may not wish to add to your life with a few blank sections to add more.

New Habit	Date Started	Description	Results
Dietary Changes			
Exercise			
Supplements			
Physiotherapy			
Chiropractic			
Massage			
Counselling			
Yoga			
Meditation			

My Journal

Use these pages to write down your thoughts. Try not to edit, use it as a way to express your concerns and feelings. No one else has to see this so I encourage you to be honest and open. I like to write down my thoughts each day before I go to bed. It helps to clear my mind of worries and to focus instead on feeling peace and gratitude. If you are wondering what to write, get started by answering these questions:

What happened today?
How do I feel about the day's events?
What are my treatment concerns?
What am I worried about?
What is the best thing that happened today?
What am I grateful for?

_____

_____

_____

_____

_____

_____

_____

_____

_____

_____

_____

_____

_____

_____

_____

_____

_____

_____

_____

_____

_____

_____

_____

_____

_____

_____

_____

_____

_____

_____

_____

_____

_____

_____

_____

_____

_____

_____

_____

_____

_____

_____

_____

_____

_____

_____

_____

_____

_____

_____

_____

_____

_____

_____

_____

_____

_____

_____

_____

_____

_____

_____

_____

_____

_____

_____

_____

_____

_____

_____

_____

_____

_____

_____

_____

_____

_____

_____

_____

_____

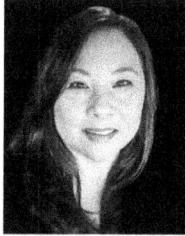

About Jo Spicer

Jo's passion for writing began as a young child growing up in Sydney, Australia. An avid reader with an overactive imagination, Jo wrote her first fiction novel at the age of 10.

Intent on developing a career with words, Jo completed her degree in Journalism and Communications at the University of Technology and embarked on a 30-year career in writing, marketing, sales, training and public speaking.

Today Jo is the author of non-fiction and fiction books in various genres including inspiration, wellness and self-development. She also writes clean romance, young adult urban fantasy and children's books.

Apart from her writing, Jo relishes good food, laughter, travel and time with family and friends. She loves creative stories in books, movies and TV series.

**For FREE giveaways, access to all of Jo's books
and updates on new releases, go to:
www.jospicer.com**

www.ingramcontent.com/pod-product-compliance
Lightning Source LLC
Chambersburg PA
CBHW062144020426
42334CB00020B/2508